The Parents' Guide to Hip Dysplasia

DEDICATION

This book is dedicated to my mom and dad,
Rosemary and Graham Lahey,
the first people I knew
who had a child with hip dysplasia.

Ordering
Trade bookstores in the U.S. and Canada please contact
Publishers Group West
1700 Fourth Street, Berkeley CA 94710
Phone: (800) 788-3123   Fax: (800) 351-5073

For bulk orders please contact
Special Sales
Hunter House Inc., PO Box 2914, Alameda CA 94501-0914
Phone: (510) 899-5041   Fax: (510) 865-4295
E-mail: sales@hunterhouse.com

Individuals can order our books by calling **(800) 266-5592**
or from our website at **www.hunterhouse.com**

THE PARENTS' GUIDE

to

HIP

DYSPLASIA

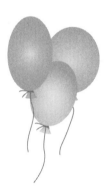

BETSY MILLER

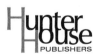

Hunter House PUBLISHERS

Hunter House Inc., Publishers
PO Box 2914
Alameda CA 94501-0914

Library of Congress Cataloging-in-Publication Data
Miller, Betsy, 1961-
The parents' guide to hip dysplasia / Betsy Miller.
pages   cm
Includes bibliographical references and index.
ISBN 978-0-89793-646-0 (pbk.) — ISBN 978-0-89793-685-9 (ebook)
1. Hip joint — Abnormalities.   2. Hip joint — Diseases.   3. Pediatric orthopedics.
I. Title.
RJ482.H55M55 2013
618.927 — dc23   2012041749

Project Credits

Cover Design: Brian Dittmar Design, Inc.

Book Production: John McKercher

Copy Editor: Amy Bauman

Indexer: Candace Hyatt

Managing Editor: Alexandra Mummery

Editorial Intern: Tu-Anh Dang-Tran

Acquisitions Coordinator: Susan Lyn McCombs

Publisher: Kiran S. Rana

Publicity Coordinator: Martha Scarpati

Special Sales Manager: Judy Hardin

Rights Coordinator: Candace Groskreutz

Customer Service Manager: Christina Sverdrup

Order Fulfillment: Washul Lakdhon

Administrator: Theresa Nelson

Computer Support: Peter Eichelberger

Printed and bound by Bang Printing, Brainerd, Minnesota
Manufactured in the United States of America

9 8 7 6 5 4 3 2 1   First Edition   13 14 15 16 17

Contents

Acknowledgments

I would like to thank my husband, Tom, and daughters, Katie and Tessa, for their understanding, support, and encouragement while I was writing this book.

Special thanks to Charles T. Price, MD, for patiently answering my many questions and for continuing to teach me about hip dysplasia treatment and to Ernest Sink, MD, for sharing his expertise in treating teens and young adults. Thank you to Kelly Ariagno, PT, and Hilary Keen, PT, C/NDT, for your insights about physical therapy in connection with hip dysplasia, and to Katherine Fan, MD, for your perspective on child and adolescent psychology.

Susan Pappas, as always, you smooth the way to make things happen, and I appreciate all of your help. Thanks to the International Hip Dysplasia Institute (IHDI) for allowing me the use of their art and X rays, and for access to the IHDI Medical Board and to Pip Mercer, Certificate IV Breastfeeding Education (Counseling and Community Education), for practical advice about breast-feeding children in hip spica casts.

Many thanks to Nancy Sanders for creating the www.hip-baby .org website, for providing ongoing support for countless parents of children with hip dysplasia, and for her practical comments and suggestions about the content of this book. Without the contributions of parents in the trenches, this book would not exist. Thank you to Jonathan Bassett, Karen Farrish, Tracy Forrester, Trent S. Heiner, Jesi Josten, Cynthia Keenan, Suzanne Lukovich, Michelle Koller, Stephanie Micke, Elle Pampinella, Heather Pass, Heather Riley, Rachel Sakaduski, Patti Sheeter, Jason Skrinak, Susette, Trina, and all the other parents out there who provide each other with practical advice and emotional support in caring for children with hip dysplasia. Thank you to the following teens for sharing your hip dysplasia experiences: Ruqayyah Abbas, Bri Keenan, Emily Marrows, and Hannah Purdy.

Rebecca Bennett, RNMS/PNP/FNP-BC; Scott Mubarak, MD; Phil Stearn, NP; Barb Brand; and Jon Wilson, CPO, were a great help in developing the previous edition of this book.

Important Note

1

Understanding
Hip Dysplasia

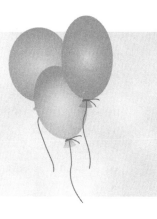

Hip dysplasia is a condition in which the top of the thighbone is not in the correct position inside the hip socket, which can affect the shape of the other bones in the hip joint. Hip dysplasia is also called *developmental dysplasia of the hip* (DDH), or *congenital dysplasia of the hip* (CDH). A baby can be born with hip dysplasia or can develop it in early life. Another condition, called unstable hips, is sometimes confused with hip dysplasia. Many babies are born with unstable hips that stabilize within two weeks after birth. With hip dysplasia, the problem persists and requires early medical treatment.

Usually, as a baby or child grows, the bones in the hip joint fit together, grow at the same rate, and stay in proportion to one another. In a child with hip dysplasia, the hip-joint structure does not fit together normally and can become progressively worse as the child's bones develop. If untreated, this can cause mobility problems as the child grows or later when he or she is an adult.

When hip dysplasia occurs, it is important to understand that a child's hips formed this way on their own. The problem was not caused by an injury. In fact, babies with hip dysplasia typically do not have hip pain, even if their hips are dislocated. Very young babies are not yet bearing weight on their hip joints by crawling or walking. Even when they reach the crawling and walking stages, these children often have no hip pain because they are still small and light. In severe cases of hip dysplasia, a baby or child can experience pain if the thighbone and the bone of the hip socket rub together. This is called "bone on bone" contact and is rare.

There is no known way to predict hip dysplasia or to prevent it from occurring, but there are certain practices that can be followed to try and reduce the incidence of hip dysplasia such as hip-healthy swaddling. Though there are different ways to treat hip dysplasia, the goal in each case is to reposition the hip joint so that it can grow correctly.

Hip-Joint Structure

Since the hip joints are hidden inside the body, most people do not think much about how they work. A hip joint is a ball-and-socket joint. The top of the thighbone (femur) is round, like a ball, and is called the femoral head. It fits deep inside the hip socket, which is called the acetabulum. Cartilage cushions the inside of the joint, and a rim of soft tissue called the labrum surrounds the joint, adding extra support. Figure 1 shows a normal hip joint for a baby.

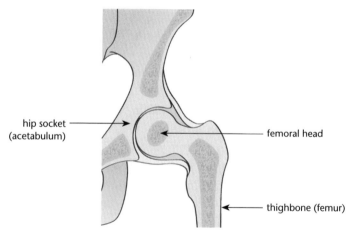

hip socket (acetabulum) — femoral head — thighbone (femur)

FIGURE 1. A normal hip joint for a young baby

The following sections explain common problems that occur with hip dysplasia.

◉ *The Top of the Thighbone (Femoral Head)*
Is in the Wrong Position

When the femoral head is in the wrong position, the hip joint cannot work normally. The hip can be unstable, subluxated (partially dislocated), or dislocated.

Unstable Hip

The femoral head can move out of the hip socket. In some cases, this happens when the doctor examines the child's hips. In other cases, it happens when the child is asleep or very relaxed.

Subluxated Hip

The femoral head is only partially in contact with the hip socket instead of completely in contact with it (see Figure 2). This happens if the hip socket is the wrong shape (malformed) and/or if the femoral head is malformed. If untreated, subluxation can eventually lead to disability and early arthritis as the hip joint wears out.

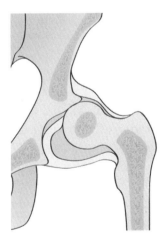

FIGURE 2. A subluxated hip, a condition in which the femoral head is partially inside the hip socket.

Dislocated Hip

The femoral head is outside the hip socket (see Figure 3 on the next page). A hip can be dislocated at birth, or it can dislocate when the child is a little older—perhaps at a year or eighteen months old. If a baby is born with dislocated hips on both sides, the problem might not show up during the newborn hip exam. Without an ultrasound or X ray, the problem could be hard to see until the baby gets older.

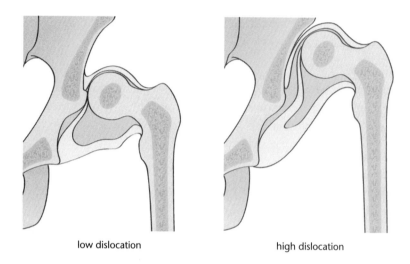

low dislocation   high dislocation

FIGURES 3A AND 3B. Each of these illustrations shows a dislocated hip, which means the femoral head is outside the hip socket.

● The Bones in the Hip Joint Are the Wrong Shape (Malformed)

When the hip socket (acetabulum) and the ball at the top of the thighbone (femoral head) are the wrong shape, it is not possible for the hip joint to work normally.

With hip dysplasia, the hip socket is often shallower than usual. Sometimes it is described as having a saucer shape instead of a cup shape. This means that the ball at the femoral head cannot fit inside the hip socket in a normal position. Doctors treat the shallow hip socket as early as possible while the baby's joints are still developing. Treatment positions the femoral head in the best alignment to encourage the hip socket to gradually deepen.

If the shallow hip socket is not treated, it affects the shape of the femoral head. As a child grows, the femoral head molds to the hip socket, becoming larger than normal. If this occurs, the femoral head is too large to fit inside a normal hip socket, which makes the hip dysplasia harder to correct.

Risk Factors

It has been found that the practice of tightly swaddling babies with their legs straight increases the incidence of hip dysplasia, but there is no known way to prevent all cases of hip dysplasia. If hip dysplasia is treated early, then it can be corrected. Though many people have never heard of hip dysplasia, it is surprisingly common. About 1 in 1,000 babies have this condition. It is more common for children who have the following risk factors.

⬤ Family History

Hip dysplasia runs in families. If a child is born with hip dysplasia, the risk of a sibling also having hip dysplasia is 6 percent (1 in 17). If an adult has hip dysplasia, the risk of his or her child having hip dysplasia is 12 percent (1 in 8). If a parent and a child have hip dysplasia, the risk that the next child will have hip dysplasia is 36 percent (1 in 3).[1]

Often when a child is diagnosed, relatives remember other family members who had hip trouble, though it might not have occurred until middle age. This can be due to undiagnosed and/or untreated cases of hip dysplasia. The hip dysplasia was mild enough for the person to manage in childhood and early adulthood. As the person aged, osteoarthritis occurred. In this case, family history may include hip replacement surgery before age sixty. If your family has a history of hip problems, be sure to tell your child's doctor.

⬤ Gender

Hip dysplasia occurs in girls nine times more often than in boys. This is thought to be due to the influence of a mother's hormones before the baby is born. Female babies might be sensitive to a hormone called relaxin, which pregnant women produce. Relaxin causes a woman's ligaments to loosen before childbirth and is also thought to cause the baby's ligaments to loosen before birth.

⬤ Firstborn, Breech, Large Babies, or Twins

The position of the baby in the womb and crowding in the womb increase the risk of babies having this condition. Crowding is more likely to occur for firstborn babies, twins, and for large babies. The breech position increases a baby's risk of conditions, such as positional plagiocephaly (head shape) and hip dysplasia that are associated with the baby's position inside the womb. These are sometimes referred to as "packaging" problems.

● Left Hip

Before birth, toward the end of the pregnancy, a baby typically lies head down in the uterus, which positions the left hip near the mother's spine. This limits movement of the left hip, which could be why this hip is more likely to have hip dysplasia.

● Straight-Legged Swaddling

Swaddling babies so that their legs are straight and close together has been shown to increase the risk of hip dysplasia. To avoid this risk, it is best to use hip-healthy swaddling. For more information, see "Hip-Healthy Swaddling" below.

Reducing the Risk for Babies

How a baby is swaddled or carried affects the incidence of hip dysplasia. This section explains some best practices that can be used for all babies to promote hip health and to reduce the number of babies who develop hip dysplasia. At this time, it is not possible to prevent all cases of hip dysplasia.

● Hip-Healthy Swaddling

Many young babies like to be swaddled. It's fine to swaddle your baby, but make sure that you leave enough room for your baby's legs to move naturally. You can swaddle your baby with a blanket or with a sleep sack product such as the HALO SleepSack Swaddle.

To swaddle your baby with a blanket:

* Lay the blanket flat and place the baby onto the blanket on his or her back.

* Gently move one arm down and wrap the blanket around the baby's arm.

* Gently move the baby's other arm down and wrap it with the blanket.

* Check to make sure that the baby's legs are relaxed and that his or her knees can easily bend (see Figure 4).

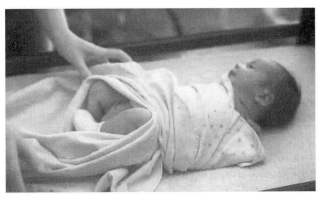

FIGURE 4. It is important to leave enough room for the baby's legs to move naturally.

* Cover the baby's legs loosely, and tuck the blanket under the baby (see Figure 5).

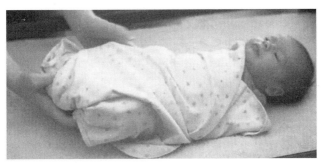

FIGURE 5. The baby can kick, but his arms are snugly wrapped, which is calming.

* When swaddling your baby with a sleep sack, make sure to leave plenty of room at the bottom of the sack for the baby's legs to move (see Figures 4 and 5). Then follow the instructions that came with your product. Figure 6 on the next page shows an example.

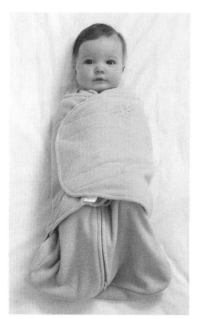

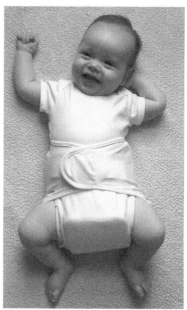

FIGURE 6. HALO SleepSack Swaddle *(Photo courtesy of HALO Innovations, Inc.)*

FIGURE 7. HALO Healthy Hips Diaper Cover *(Photo courtesy of HALO Innovations, Inc.)*

● *Double or Triple Diapering*

Your doctor might tell you to double or triple diaper your baby until she can fit the Pavlik harness or a brace. This can help keep the hips in a healthy position and encourage better hip-joint development. HALO Innovations makes a diaper cover that was specifically developed for babies with loose hips.

● *Baby Carrying*

There are a number of slings, wraps, and baby carriers available (see Figures 8 and 9 for examples). When choosing to carry a baby, make sure that the baby is supported and that the legs can bend in a natural position.

The diagram in Figure 10 shows how carrying a baby with the right support helps keep the hip joints aligned.

If a baby is carried without support for the hips and with the legs close together, the hip joint is less stable. It is more likely that the hip joint can move out of alignment as shown in the diagram in Figure 11.

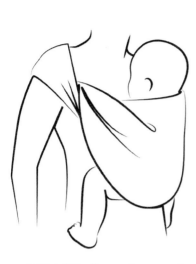

FIGURE 8. This sling carrier supports the baby's legs and holds the hips in a healthy position.

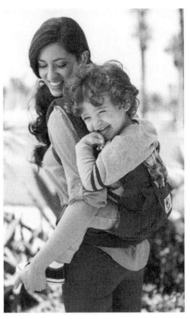

FIGURE 9. This baby carrier supports the child's legs and holds the hips in a healthy position. *(Photo provided by ERGObaby.com)*

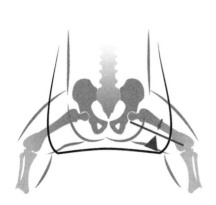

FIGURE 10. For each hip, the ball at the top of the thighbone (the femoral head) is inside the hip socket.

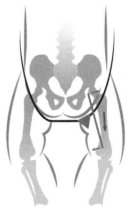

The femoral heads are coming out of the hip sockets.

FIGURE 11. This baby's hips have moved out of alignment.

It's okay if your baby's legs are sometimes in the position shown in Figure 11 on the previous page. For instance, your baby's legs might look like this when he or she is lying down, or as you pick him or her up to be carried. The stress on the hips occurs only when babies are carried this way for an extended period of time.

● Car Seats

While all car seats are designed to protect babies and children who are riding in a car, they vary in how much room is allotted for a baby's legs and hips. It is best to use a car seat that is wide enough at the bottom so that the baby's legs are in a natural position.

Avoid car seats that are narrow at the bottom. When sitting in them, the baby's legs are positioned too close together, which isn't good for the hips.

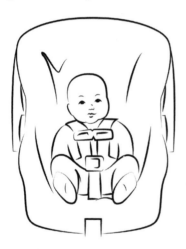 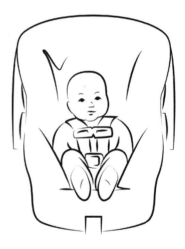

FIGURE 12. In this car seat, the baby's legs are in a healthy position.

FIGURE 13. This style of car seat is not recommended because the seat is too narrow.

What Happens If Hip Dysplasia Is Not Treated?

In the long run, hip dysplasia can cause uneven leg lengths, limping, and hip clicks. It can also cause problems with the structure of the hip joint, such as bones growing into the wrong shape, which can be seen in ultrasounds or X rays. As mentioned earlier in this chapter, a normal hip-socket shape is deep like a cup; with hip dysplasia, the hip socket can become shallow like a saucer.

Over the course of a lifetime, wear and tear occur in the cartilage inside the joints of the human body. The hip joints are no exception. For people with hip dysplasia, the hip cartilage tends to wear out unevenly and at an earlier age than usual. Because the bones in the hip joint are not the ideal shape, the hip joint carries its load unevenly. Some areas of cartilage can wear out faster than others, resulting in arthritis.

The labrum is a rim of soft tissue that surrounds each hip joint. People with hip dysplasia often have larger labrums than usual. The labrums develop this way to compensate for the shallow hip sockets. This lends some stability to the joint, but the labrum is not as strong as bone. The stress of movement and support can cause the labrum to tear in adolescence or adulthood. This is called a labral tear.

When a person has untreated hip dysplasia, how the hip joint changes over time depends on how severe the problem is. Some common conditions associated with hip dysplasia are described here.

Osteoarthritis

With hip dysplasia, cartilage in the hip joint wears out unevenly, which leads to osteoarthritis. Depending on how severe the problem is, people with untreated hip dysplasia may begin to experience hip pain in their thirties or forties. In very severe cases, teenagers and young adults can develop arthritis.

Hip Labral Tear

This rim of cartilage is more susceptible to tearing in people with hip dysplasia. Especially when the hip socket is shallow, as it can be with this condition, the bones in the hip joint do not offer enough support for this soft tissue.

Limping and Knee Problems

If only one hip is affected by hip dysplasia, the person limps. The legs can be different lengths. The knee can become deformed due to the uneven mechanics within the hip joint. The knee might carry a heavier than usual load to compensate for the hip-joint structure, and knee pain can result.

● Difficulty Walking or Running

When the bones in the hip joint are not positioned correctly or are malformed, they do not support the load of the joint evenly. Muscles must work extra hard to compensate for the bone structure. These muscles get tired faster than usual, and this can cause difficulty walking or running.

● Scoliosis (a Curved Spine)

Scoliosis can occur if one hip has hip dysplasia or is dislocated and one hip is higher than the other. Think about standing with one shoe on and one shoe off. If the pelvis is always tilted when a child stands, in some cases the spine will compensate by curving.

● False Hip Sockets

When both hips are dislocated, the child has a waddling gait (the hip swings from side to side). Back pain can develop. One of the most severe complications that can occur is if false hip sockets develop in the wrong place. If left untreated, the sockets that the child was born with can gradually fill in with bone so that it is no longer possible for the top of the thighbones to be aligned correctly. This condition leads to arthritis in the long run.

Hip Dysplasia Can Be Treated, but Not All Cases Can Be Prevented

It is only natural to ask why a baby or young child has a condition like hip dysplasia. Many parents worry that they did something to cause it or wonder if they could have prevented it in some way. Though the risk factors listed in the previous section make it more likely that a person will have hip dysplasia, it cannot be predicted or prevented. It isn't anyone's fault, but you can do things to help your child if he or she has it.

With early medical treatment, hip dysplasia can be corrected. Doctors check for hip dysplasia when they examine babies and young children. Hip exams are done for newborns and during regular checkups. If the doctor suspects hip dysplasia, or if a baby is at risk, ultrasounds or X rays are done. Babies and children found to have hip dysplasia are referred to pediatric orthopedic doctors. The next chapter explains how doctors check for hip dysplasia and how ultrasounds and X rays are used to better understand the structure of the hip joint.

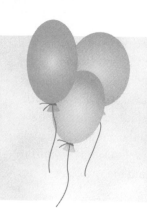

2

Checking for
Hip Dysplasia

When doctors examine babies and children at birth and at well-baby checkups, they routinely check the hips. If a hip problem is suspected, then ultrasound imaging or X rays are used to reveal the structure of the hip joint, and the baby or child is seen by a pediatric orthopedic doctor. These doctors have special training to diagnose and treat bone and joint problems in babies and children. This chapter describes hip exams and the ultrasounds and X rays that doctors use to check for hip dysplasia.

Some cases of hip dysplasia are harder to spot than others. If both hips are affected (bilateral), and the baby is not thought to be at risk for hip dysplasia, the problem might not be obvious when the baby is very young. When I was a baby, my mother noticed that something was not quite right about my hips. She took me to the doctor, and I was diagnosed with bilateral hip dysplasia. I have two older brothers with no hip problems, and our family did not have any risk factors.

Another significant reason why hip dysplasia can be hard to spot is that it can develop as a child grows. Previously, it was believed that all cases of hip dysplasia could be detected in infancy. This has turned out not to be the case. A report from Norway, where medical personnel screen all babies for hip dysplasia, showed that the majority of adults under forty who needed total hip replacements due to hip dysplasia had been examined as babies and at that time were found to have normal hips. This means that the hip dysplasia developed after the babies were first examined. Some cases of older children having dislocated hips can be attributed to tightly swaddling the babies with their legs straight, but many cases can have other causes as well.

Hip Exams for Young Babies (Newborn to Four Months of Age)

Babies' hips are examined soon after birth and during routine check-ups. Doctors check to see if the hips are unstable, if hip dysplasia is present, or if the hips are dislocated. The doctor moves the baby's legs to see how easily the legs move apart and also moves the hips and legs in specific ways to see if there is anything unusual in the movement that might indicate a problem. Standard exams that doctors use are called the Ortolani test, the Galeazzi test, and the Barlow's test. Each test takes only a few minutes and does not hurt the baby. The tests are described in the following sections.

● The Ortolani Test for Newborns

The Ortolani test checks to see if the baby's hip joints are dislocatable (the top of the thighbone can slide in and out of the hip socket). This test does not work for an older baby. If an older baby has a dislocated hip, it might not be able to go back into the hip socket.

During this test, the doctor puts the baby's legs in a frog-leg position and then moves the legs apart. If a hip is dislocatable, the doctor hears a clunking sound at the same time that he or she feels the top of the thighbone go into the hip socket. Figure 14 shows a positive Ortolani test.

Some normal hips click or snap in daily life or during this test. These sounds alone do not mean that a baby's hip is dislocatable.

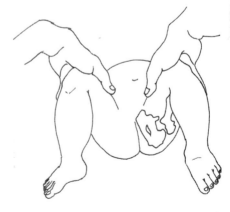

FIGURE 14. A sample Ortolani test. The result shown is positive for a dislocatable hip.

● *The Barlow's Test*

This test also is used to see if a baby's hip easily dislocates. A hip that easily dislocates is unstable. Less than 2 percent of babies have a positive result with this test. Most of these unstable hips stabilize on their own without treatment; 60 percent stabilize within one month, and 88 percent stabilize within two months.

The hips are checked one at a time. The doctor places his hands over the baby's hipbones and holds one leg steady. The leg on the side that is being examined is moved outward. If the top of the thighbone moves out of the hip joint and then slides back in, the doctor can feel it. A positive result means the hip can be dislocated. Figure 15 shows a positive Barlow's test.

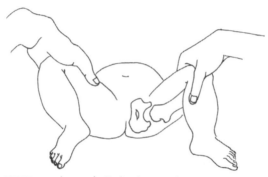

FIGURE 15. A sample Barlow's test. The result shown is positive for a dislocatable hip.

● *The Galeazzi Test*

This test checks for one dislocated hip, which makes one leg look longer than the other. When a hip is dislocated, the ball at the top of the thighbone (femoral head) is completely outside the hip socket.

If the baby has bilateral hip dysplasia (both sides are affected) or both of the baby's hips are dislocated, then the doctor might not be able to tell that there is a problem from the Galeazzi test. In these situations, the legs could be the same length.

During the exam, the baby is placed flat on her back. The doctor bends the baby's hips and knees so that the baby's feet are flat. If the knees are not the same height, this is a positive result for one hip. A positive result means that the baby could have a dislocated hip or a short thighbone (femur) on one side. Figure 16 shows a child with a positive Galeazzi test.

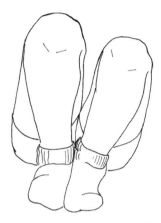

FIGURE 16. A sample Galeazzi test. The result shown is positive for a dislocated hip.

Note: During everyday activities such as a diaper change at home, a baby's legs could be in this position. A parent or caretaker might notice that the baby's legs appear to be different lengths. If you notice this problem, notify your child's doctor.

● *Exam Results for Young Babies*
Results of the hip exam can be negative, mixed, or positive:

Negative
The hips showed no problems.

Mixed
Sometimes the results are mixed, or minor symptoms are present that could either be due to unstable hips that will resolve without treatment or to hip dysplasia. If the results are unclear, the doctor will recommend an ultrasound or X rays to get more information about the structure of the hip joint.

Positive
A positive result means that the child has hip dysplasia.

Many newborn babies have unstable hips. Most become stable on their own within the first two weeks after birth. Newborns with unstable or dislocated hips might be reexamined when they are two weeks old to see if the problem persists. If the baby is two weeks of age or older and the problem is still occurring, the baby usually is referred to a pediatric orthopedic doctor. A pediatric orthopedic doctor specializes in medical problems involving bones and joints in children.

Hip Exams for Children and Teens

As with a baby, if a child or teen is thought to have hip dysplasia, he or she also should be referred to a pediatric orthopedic doctor. This is advised even for teens who are adult size. A pediatric orthopedic doctor specializes in medical problems involving bones and joints in children.

As with babies, the doctor looks for signs of a hip problem: uneven leg lengths, a limp, an unusual gait, a clicking sound when the hips are moved in a specific way during the exam. The doctor observes the child's stance and gait. Here are some things the doctor looks for:

* When standing, are the feet in an unusual position? For example, are they turned very far outward or very far inward?

* Does one leg appear to be longer? For example, does the child have one foot flat on the ground and the other on tiptoe?

* Is the spine straight, or is it curved to one side?

* Does the child limp?

* Does the child walk with a waddling gait (making the hips swing from side to side)?

These problems can be associated with hip dysplasia or with other orthopedic conditions. In addition to an exam, X rays are used to reveal the structure of the hip joint.

The doctor checks the range of motion of the hip and tests for impingement. Femoral acetabular impingement (FAI) has to do with how the bones in the hip joint are shaped. It is not usually caused by hip dysplasia, but it can cause hip pain. The doctor also tests for muscle strength and presses on various areas to see if any particular spots are tender. The exam for a teen is pretty much the same whether or not he or she has had hip surgery in the past. With teens, the doctor might also check for signs of a torn labrum.

● Exam Results for Children or Teens

Children and teens may be examined for hip dysplasia because they were diagnosed and treated when they were younger or because they have started to have symptoms that could be caused by hip dysplasia. Hip dysplasia presents differently in individuals and can range from mild to severe. The degree of hip dysplasia can also change as a child grows and develops, which is why it is referred to as developmental dysplasia of the hip.

Hip dysplasia can be associated with larger than usual labrums (the rim of cartilage that surrounds the hip joint and helps stabilize it) in the hip joint. When the hip sockets are shallow, the larger labrum adds some extra support to the joint. In teens or adults, the stress of movement combined with the weight of an adult-size or nearly adult-size body, can result in a torn labrum (see Figure 17).

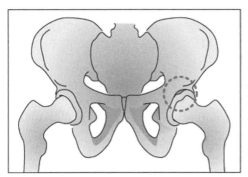 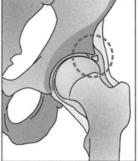

FIGURE 17. This example shows a hip joint with a tear in the labrum (the cartilage that surrounds the hip joint).

A torn labrum is a painful injury that can cause a catching sensation in the joint when it is moved in a particular way. When the structure of the hip joint is the reason for the torn labrum, the teen might need surgery to realign the hip joint and repair the tear at the same time. Note that people without hip dysplasia can also tear labrums, typically during intense sports activity, in which case the cause and treatment can be different.

Ultrasound for Young Babies

Ultrasound uses high-frequency sound waves to reveal organs or structures inside the body. Usually babies need an ultrasound only if the doctor wants to check for a problem such as hip dysplasia. If a doctor suspects hip dysplasia, or if a young baby is at risk, the American Academy of Pediatrics (AAP) recommends a hip ultrasound.

Since a new baby's bones are not solid enough to show up clearly on an X rays, ultrasound is usually preferred for babies from birth to four months of age. Some doctors, however, use X rays for babies as young as three months. Ultrasound reveals more about the hip joint than the doctor can determine from a physical exam. In some cases, it might uncover a problem that cannot be detected in a physical exam. It can also show that the child's hips are fine.

On the ultrasound image, the doctor measures the angles of the hip joint. The angle that is most often referred to in connection with hip dysplasia is the alpha angle. The alpha angle is considered normal if it is more than 60 degrees. An alpha angle from 43 to 60 degrees indicates mild hip dysplasia. An alpha angle of less than 43 degrees is associated with severe hip dysplasia.

Ultrasound does not hurt, but many babies dislike the experience. Be prepared for crying that stops as soon as the ultrasound is over. The ultrasound process is the same for babies as it is for adults. An ultrasound technologist or radiologist puts clear gel on the baby's hip area and presses a handheld device called a transducer against each hip. The person doing the ultrasound might need to move the baby's legs into specific positions to get clear images of the hip joints.

During the ultrasound exam, the hip is checked for stability in the same way as in a Barlow's test (see "The Barlow's Test" on page 16), but the ultrasound image is used to see if the hip is unstable instead of relying on only what the doctor can feel. Many babies have slightly loose hips, which can make findings of a physical exam difficult to interpret. The ultrasound images typically can show how far out of the socket the hip will move. This depends on how hard the examiner pushes. More than 50 percent of the ball at the top of the thighbone should stay inside the socket. When the number is less than 45 percent, then the hip is deemed unstable. Some instability in a six-week-old infant is not uncommon. Sometimes this is treated, and sometimes it is checked again with another ultrasound at the age of three months.

● Ultrasound Graf Scale Hip Types

One method that doctors use to interpret an infant hip ultrasound is the Graf scale, which classifies hips into Type I through Type IV.

Type 1

A Type I hip indicates a normal hip structure. The hip socket is well formed, and the top of the thighbone (femoral head) is in the correct position within the hip socket.

Type II

Type II hips can be seen in babies younger than three months or in older babies with mild hip dysplasia. In this case, the hip socket is shallow and has a rounded rim.

Type III

With a Type III hip, the hip socket is very shallow, and the top of the thighbone (femoral head) is out of position. This hip is said to be subluxated, which means that the femoral head is only partially in contact with the hip socket.

Type IV

In a Type IV hip, the ball at the top of the thighbone (femoral head) is outside the hip socket (dislocated) and the hip socket is flat. In addition to the Graf-scale type, dislocated hips can be said to have high dislocation or low dislocation. See Figures 3A and 3B on page 4 for illustrations of each of these conditions.

X Rays

X rays are a form of electromagnetic radiation. In a health-care setting, a machine sends X rays through the body, and a computer or special film records the images that are created. X rays show the doctor the shape and position of the bones in the hip joints. This helps the doctor diagnose hip dysplasia and determine which treatment is best. Babies younger than three or four months usually have ultrasounds because their bones are not solid enough to show up well on X rays (see "Ultrasound for Young Babies" on page 20).

When a baby is diagnosed with hip dysplasia, X rays are taken periodically by a health-care worker such as a medical radiation technologist to monitor the development of the hip joints. Medical personnel use a dose of radiation that is as low as is reasonably achievable (ALARA). Typically, the amount of radiation used is similar to what you would get when flying in an airplane for two hours. If your child needs X rays, go to an X-ray facility experienced in pediatrics. The equipment there is calibrated for babies and children.

For children who need hip surgery, additional X rays called arthrograms are taken. An arthrogram is an X ray of a joint that has had special dye injected into it. For more information, see "Arthography (Arthrogram)" on the next page. In some cases, computed tomography (CT) or magnetic resonance imaging (MRI) is used to provide more information about a joint.

● Gonad Shielding

Gonad shielding is the practice of putting small, lead shields over the ovaries or testes when X rays are taken of the pelvic area. For many years, this was recommended because ovaries and testes are sensitive to radiation. A recent study[2] of pelvic X rays of children found that for girls, the shields were placed incorrectly so that 91 percent of the time they did not actually cover the ovaries. For boys, the shields were placed incorrectly 66 percent of the time. The same study measured the radiation exposure with modern X-ray equipment and found the dosage to be very small (from 0.008 to 0.098 mSv). The study concluded that it might be better to stop using gonad shielding.

In the context of hip dysplasia, one reason why it can be difficult to place the shields is that the shields might block the hip joint. If the shields are in the wrong place, then an extra X ray must be taken. In this case it would have been better not to use the shields. In some cases if a child is wearing a cast, the curve of the cast makes the shields slip out of position.

Feel free to ask about gonad shielding, as different facilities might have different policies. If you are worried about X rays, discuss the topic with your child's doctor.

● Arthrogram (Arthrography)

An arthrogram, also called an arthrography, is an X ray taken after a special dye is injected into a joint. This lets the doctor see the tendons, ligaments, muscles, cartilage, and the joint lining. These areas, also called soft tissues, do not show up well on a regular X ray. An arthrogram in a child requires anesthesia.

For children with hip dysplasia, arthrography is often done with a reduction (putting the femoral head into the hip socket) or after a cast is put on or changed. An arthrogram before a reduction gives the doctor a clearer picture of the joint structure than an X ray. After the reduction is done and the child is in a cast, the doctor does an arthrogram to make sure that the femoral head is in the right place in the hip socket.

● Interpreting X Rays

Figure 18 on the next page shows the information about hip-joint structure that an X ray reveals. The doctor draws lines onto the X ray to show how the ball at the top of the thighbone (femoral head) interacts with the hip socket (acetabulum). The first lines are vertical and horizontal and are similar to compass lines. The vertical line (north/south) is called Perkin's line. The horizontal line (east/west) is called Hilgenreiner's line.

Perkin's Line

A vertical line is drawn at the outside edge of each hip socket. With a normal hip, the femoral head is inside this line (closer to the center of the body than to the outside edge of the hip socket).

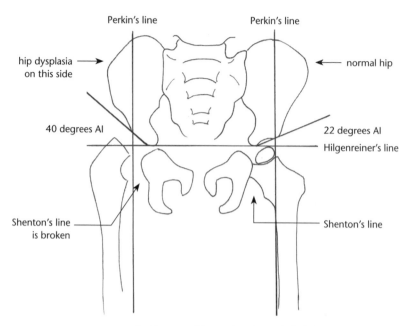

FIGURE 18. An illustrated X ray showing a baby's hip structure at the age of eight months.

Hilgenreiner's Line

This is a horizontal line drawn at the top of the triradiate cartilages, a specific part of the hip bone that doctors can easily identify. With a normal hip, the femoral head is below this line.

Acetabular Index (AI)

The acetabular index is the angle, marked by a line drawn on an X ray, from the bottom of the pelvis to the outer edge of the socket and Hilgenreiner's line. The measurement of this angle changes in all babies and children as they grow. Crawling, walking, and weight-bearing exercise cause the hip sockets to become deeper as the child grows. With normal hips, the AI is within a specified range depending on the age of the child. For example, an AI under 30 is normal for a one-year-old child. The goal in hip dysplasia treatment is to encourage the hip sockets to develop within the normal range. For children with hip dysplasia, even after successful treatment, the AI might be different for each hip but still within the normal range.

Note: Some doctors do not discuss the AI. If a child has a severe dislocation, there might not be an AI because the femoral head is up high and far away from the hip socket.

Shenton's Line

In normal hips, a smooth arc can be drawn between the obturator foramen (sit bones) and the femoral neck (the part of the thighbone just below the ball at the top). This is called Shenton's line. If the thighbone is out of position, sometimes it is not possible to draw this line. Figure 18 shows Shenton's line both intact and broken.

Percent Coverage

Percent coverage is sometimes given together with the AI. This is the amount of coverage that the hip socket provides for the femoral head. The percent coverage can increase as the baby grows and develops. Here is an example of how one hospital schedules an ultrasound based on the percent coverage of an ultrasound taken of a baby at six weeks of age:

* Fifty percent coverage or higher is normal.

* Forty to 50 percent coverage with a normal exam: Schedule an ultrasound when the baby is four months old.

* Less than 40 percent coverage with a normal exam: Schedule an ultrasound when the baby is ten weeks old.

CE Angle

The CE angle, also called the CE angle of Wiberg, is used to assess hip structure for adults and children over the age of five. To get the CE angle, the doctor draws a line on the X ray from the center of the femoral head to the outside edge of the top of the hip socket. She or he then draws a second vertical line through the center of the femoral head. The angle formed by the intersection of those lines is the CE angle. A CE angle over 25 degrees is considered normal; a hip with severe hip dysplasia may have a CE angle of less than 20 degrees.

● *Variations in X-Ray Results*

The pediatric orthopedic doctor monitors the X-ray results and adjusts treatment as needed based on the child's progress. If several X rays are taken at the same time and the hips look good in one position but not another, it could mean that the hips can move within the hip sockets. It could also mean the child was twisted, and the X ray might not be accurate. Different doctors can have varied interpretations of the same X ray depending on their knowledge of childhood hip dysplasia. That is why it is best to go to a pediatric orthopedic doctor to interpret the X rays.

Computed Tomography (CT)

A computed tomography exam, or CT, is a special type of X ray that provides more detail than a standard X ray does. During the CT, the X-ray beam moves around the body so that images can be seen from many angles. The final images show "slices" of the area being scanned. The equipment looks like a large box with a round hole in the side. The X-ray scanner is built into the equipment and is controlled by a health-care worker who is in the next room and can see the child and equipment through a window. Some facilities let a parent stay with a child while the equipment is being set up. The child lies on a table that moves in and out of the scanner. The CT is sent to a computer located in a different room, where it is checked by a radiologist. Sometimes a CT is done after surgery to confirm the position of the femoral head in the hip socket.

CT scans use X rays, and the dose is higher than a standard X ray. During a CT scan, the exposure is lowered as much as possible for children or babies, and as few "slices" as possible are done. Ask your child's doctor to recommend a facility that has experience working with children so that the child's exposure is minimized.

Magnetic Resonance Imaging (MRI)

Magnetic resonance imaging (MRI) does not use X rays. It uses a strong magnetic field and radio waves to create images of tissues. This allows the doctor see the ligaments, muscles, joint surface, and tendons (also called soft tissue) around a joint much more clearly than on an X ray. Babies and children are put to sleep with anesthesia if they need an MRI so that they stay still and the images are clear. In some situations, the doctor might recommend an MRI with contrast (dye) or using a high-resolution MRI machine to reveal more detail about the joint. Not all facilities have the highest resolution machines. If dye is used, a local anesthetic is injected into the hip joint first and then the contrast material is injected. For instance, a teen who is thought to have a tear in the labrum (the soft rim of cartilage that surrounds the hip joint) might have a high-resolution MRI or an MRI with contrast.

Several types of MRI equipment are used. Traditionally, MRI equipment has been long and narrow, but newer designs with more open sides are sometimes used. Depending on the number of images needed, the MRI can take from 15 to 45 minutes to complete.

Because MRI does not use X rays, there is no concern about radiation exposure. The main safety concern with MRI is that the strong magnets can cause metal objects to move very quickly, which could injure someone. Before an MRI, medical personnel use questionnaires and follow standard procedures to keep metal objects out of the room.

Your Child's Diagnosis

Based on the results of the hip exam and an ultrasound or X rays, the pediatric orthopedic doctor can tell if the baby or child has hip dysplasia. Finding out that your child has hip dysplasia can be a shock, and many parents of children diagnosed with the condition have similar reactions. As one mother from the Hip-baby online support group says: "I was so scared and cried nonstop. It is normal. The fear of the unknown is worse than the reality [of treatment]. It really is."

● Hip-Baby Discussion Group

Some parents have doubts about the diagnosis or treatment. If you feel this way, get a second, or even a third, opinion. Finding a doctor you are comfortable with is important (see "Choosing a Pediatric Orthopedic Doctor" on page 34). If your child was diagnosed late, you might be angry that the hip dysplasia was not caught at a younger age. One mother of a child with a severe case of hip dysplasia offers these suggestions:

Anger can be useful if you use it in a constructive way, such as advo-cating for your child. Bitterness just gets in the way. Try to stop thinking about what might have been and to be optimistic about the outcome. It might take you some time but find the strength to be positive for the sake of your child.   [HEATHER]

One parent has this to say about what helped their family through the experience:

From the time my daughter was diagnosed with hip dysplasia until I was able to reach out and get other parents' perspective and ex-perience, I was a total mess. My mind raced in a hundred different directions, and I kept coming up with new and different questions with no clear answers. Once I was able to speak to other parents [who had gone] through a similar experience, a lot of my fears and concerns were resolved. My wife and I were extremely lucky to have such a strong little girl. Samantha was unbelievable through the whole process—but just knowing others have gone through this made things just a little easier.

If I could recommend anything to those who have just had their child diagnosed, I would suggest brainstorming as many questions as possible and make sure you get these answered by not only the doctors but also parents who have made the similar journey you are about to face. The more information and facts you have, the less fear and concern you will have of the unknown. I would also say not to be stubborn and take any offers for assistance. We have amazing family and friends who went out of their way to make our situation a little more bearable and for that I would like to thank them from the bottom of my heart!   [JASON]

3

Developing a
Treatment Plan

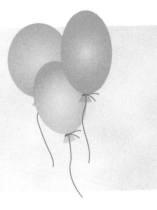

This chapter explains treatment for hip dysplasia, how doctors describe a hip dysplasia diagnosis, and medical conditions that increase the risk of hip dysplasia. It also covers the role of doctors and health-care workers and offers some basic advice about medical insurance and other types of financial support for treatment.

But first: If your child is diagnosed with hip dysplasia, take a moment to remember that he or she is exactly the same person as before the diagnosis—sweet, funny, imaginative, shy, or impossible to please. The difference is that now you know your child needs some extra help. How much extra help? Hip dysplasia can vary from mild to severe.

Take your child to an expert—a pediatric orthopedic doctor who has experience with hip dysplasia. These doctors have special training to diagnose and treat bone or joint problems in babies and children. A regular orthopedic doctor does not have this special training about the details of how bones and joints change and grow in a baby or young child. The pediatric orthopedic doctor looks at the ultrasound or X rays and examines the child. Then the doctor diagnoses the child and chooses the best treatment.

Since hip dysplasia can run in families, having a child diagnosed with hip dysplasia sometimes causes parents to pay more attention to their own hip health. Although a number of different medical conditions can cause pain in the hip area, if you think you might have undiagnosed hip dysplasia, it is best to check with your doctor. See "Adult Treatment" on page 116.

Treatments for Hip Dysplasia

The goal of treatment is for your child to have stable hips with the best possible structure. In a healthy hip, the ball at the top of the thighbone (femoral head) must be in the hip socket in the correct position. In severe cases in which a baby did not develop hip sockets, the femoral heads are put into the best position to encourage hip sockets to develop. How the doctor treats your child depends on the extent of the problem in the hip joint, and treatment might change as your child grows and develops.

If you have a baby or young child, your doctor might have you temporarily double diaper or triple diaper your child to keep his or her legs apart until treatment begins.

The following treatments are recommended for hip dysplasia:

* Pavlik harness, a soft brace for babies
* hip abduction brace for a baby or young child
* reduction surgery and a cast for a baby
* osteotomy surgery, which may be followed by a cast
* total hip replacement (THR) surgery, which is used very rarely for teens who have finished growing

● Adolescent Soft Tissue Irritation or Pain

Soft tissue refers to the muscles, tendons, ligaments, cartilage, and other parts of the joint besides the bones. Because teens are close to the size and weight of adults, prior to surgical treatment they might experience some of the same problems with the soft tissue in their hips that are seen in adults with hip dysplasia. Your teen's doctor develops a treatment plan to manage inflammation or pain if your teen is experiencing either. Pain and inflammation are symptoms that can be caused by problems in the structure of the hip joint, such as bursitis or a torn labrum. Bursitis is irritation of the bursa, a soft, fluid-filled sac that acts like a cushion between the joint surfaces. The labrum is that soft rim of cartilage that surrounds the joint. Your teen might take over-the-counter or prescription pain relief medicine for pain the hip is causing. In some cases, a steroid injection can give temporary relief to soft tissue irritation, but it cannot correct the hip dysplasia itself. And because too many injections can be harmful, doctors are cautious about this treatment.

Coping with Your Child's Treatment

Though you might be concerned about treatment, bear in mind that children are resilient. Make the decisions that you believe to be in your child's best interest.

Even when you and your doctor have chosen a path of treatment, aspects of the process will still be unsettling. For instance, not knowing how long treatment will take can be stressful. Some parents find that waiting to see if a treatment is working is the hardest part of having a child with hip dysplasia. And feeling sad is common. You might be especially sad the first time you see your child in a Pavlik harness or brace, or when you're facing your child's surgery. Even small things, like baby clothes that won't fit over the Pavlik harness or spica cast, can trigger these feelings. Parents of children diagnosed at a later age might feel sad if they see their child watching while others run and play. A mother from the Hip-baby online support group (www.hip-baby.org) offers this perspective:

We spend so much time telling ourselves it will be okay, she'll never remember, aren't we lucky it isn't a serious illness, that we don't take enough time to grieve for our losses. Ultimately, this, too, will pass, but in the meantime, it is a loss. You spend your entire pregnancy imagining holding your sweet baby, and I know none of my fantasies involved a cast, or brace, or harness.

[HIP-BABY DISCUSSION GROUP]

As your child goes through treatment, take the time to enjoy and admire him or her. Remember that there is more to him or her than hip dysplasia. Spend time together on some activities that are based on what the child can do rather than focusing on any temporary limitations during treatment.

Involving Adolescents in the Treatment Plan

When hip dysplasia is present in older children or adolescents, it may be due to residual hip dysplasia after early childhood treatment, or it may be due to a late diagnosis. Or if your child has Down syndrome or cerebral palsy, he or she may have developed hip dysplasia over time. It's a good idea to ask your child's doctor the following questions:

* How severe is the hip dysplasia?
* Is my child experiencing symptoms or in pain?
* If surgery is needed, can it be planned for summer so that it will have less of an impact on school?

Include teens in discussions about treatment so that they understand the reason for surgery (how surgery will improve their hip joint) and have some understanding of the recovery and rehabilitation process involved. For comments from teens who have been through surgery for hip dysplasia, see "Teen Voices" on page 164.

Teens who would like to get to know other teens and young adults with hip dysplasia might like to visit the online group Happy Hips (http://happyhips.webs.com). Two teenage girls with hip dysplasia started this group, and it has been steadily growing in size.

Communicating with Doctors

It is important to understand what your child's treatment will be, how it will help your child, and what you must do in order for the treatment to be effective.

When interacting with a doctor, you can get this information in a variety of ways. Some people like a short explanation (get to the main point, please). Others (like me) prefer to ask questions. Over the years I have talked to doctors who were happy to answer my questions and doctors who were less enthusiastic about my approach. In a perfect world, the questioners would be matched up with the happy-to-answer caregivers, and the "get to the point" people would be matched with caregivers who give the concise answers that they like. It is nice, but not always possible, to get a caregiver who matches your communication style.

Medical treatment for a baby or young child can be stressful for families. Parents sometimes disagree or argue about the cause of the hip dysplasia and the need for treatment. It might help if both parents are able to talk to the doctor and ask questions about any areas of confusion. If only one parent can visit the doctor's office, try to schedule it at a time when the other parent can phone in and join the conversation on a speaker phone or cell phone.

The following questions present information that you should learn from your doctor so that you will understand your child's treatment:

* Why is this treatment needed?

* How long does the treatment usually last?

* What would be the best possible outcome and the worst possible outcome of this treatment?

* Is my child in pain? Does he or she need pain relief now?

In most cases of hip dysplasia, the child is not in pain. However in some severe cases, the bones rub together, which is painful. If this is the case, discuss pain relief for your child. For children who need surgery, anesthesia and pain relief medicines are used.

If you do not understand your child's doctor or are uncomfortable with the care that your child is receiving, bring up the questions or problems that concern you. Some people find this difficult, but it is worth making the effort. Learn more about diagnosis and treatment or get a second opinion so that you feel comfortable with your child's treatment.

Choosing a Pediatric Orthopedic Doctor

When beginning treatment for your child's hip dysplasia, you will probably be referred to a pediatric orthopedic doctor who is in the same medical group as your child's pediatrician. Common practice in referrals varies from one location to another.

The importance of having your child seen by a pediatric orthopedic doctor is that this doctor specializes in muscle and bone problems in children. An orthopedic doctor who works with adults does not know as much about childhood hip dysplasia. Ask the doctor how many cases of hip dysplasia he or she has treated. Some have more experience than others. And if your child needs surgery, ideally it is best to seek out a doctor experienced in the type of surgery your child needs and at a hospital in which the surgery is done on a regular basis.

Some ways to find a pediatric orthopedic doctor are listed here:

* Ask your pediatrician for recommendations.

* Ask for a referral to your local children's hospital if it specializes in orthopedics.

* Search for medical groups and organizations on the Internet. See "Hip Dysplasia Websites and Organizations" on page 188.

* Check with your local Easter Seals (a nonprofit organization). This group might have a list of pediatric orthopedic doctors whom their clients use. See "Health and Medical Organizations" on page 190.

* Contact a Shriners hospital pediatric orthopedic department (associated with the Shriners organization). See "Health and Medical Organizations" on page 190.

Getting a Second Opinion

Although treatment for hip dysplasia aims for the same result in every case—to encourage the development of normal hip joints—the style of treatment varies from one doctor to another. Also, some pediatric orthopedic doctors have more experience treating hip dysplasia than others. It is a good idea to get a second opinion from another pediatric orthopedic doctor so that you feel comfortable with your child's treatment plan. Getting a second opinion will not offend the original doctor.

For example, a one-year-old who needed a reduction was seen by three pediatric orthopedic doctors. The first doctor recommended an open reduction. The second doctor wanted to try to do a closed reduction followed by a plaster cast. If that did not work, he would wait until the child was 18 months old and then do an open reduction. The third doctor was confident that a closed reduction would work and recommended a fiberglass/Gore-Tex cast to be worn for a longer period of time. This family chose to go to the third doctor, but another family might have made a different choice.

Cynthia's daughter Bri was diagnosed with hip dysplasia when she was a teenager. Bri underwent Periacetabular osteotomy (PAO) surgery. Cynthia offers this advice about interacting with doctors:

As far as the medical part of the journey goes, my top advice is to listen to your gut and keep asking questions until you get answers that make sense. If a doctor tells you something that just doesn't seem right or goes against what another doctor says, ask another doctor. In my experience, the best doctors not only have the credentials and experience behind them, but they listen carefully to your questions. I have learned that some of the smartest doctors might not have all the answers right in front of them. But they are willing to dig deeper, too. They are willing to talk to other doctors. They are open to suggestions and recommendations from other experts.

In my daughter's case, I believe her surgeons are among the best in the world. It doesn't mean they are perfect, but we trust them. They listen, they care, and there is no arrogance. It took quite awhile for us to get to them, and physically getting to them is a challenge in that they are 1,500 miles away from our home. In the end, I believe the time and effort we have made will pay off. Our hope is that when Bri goes to college next year, this will all be behind her.   [CYNTHIA]

Though Cynthia and Bri traveled for Bri's surgery, you might not need to do so. Look into medical treatment near your home first. Then, if necessary, widen your search to include other locations. Generally speaking the best outcomes for surgery tend to be associated with doctors who, on a regular basis, have experience in the specific surgery and hospitals at which that surgery is performed.

Medical Records

You can ask for a copy of your child's medical records, including X rays, and MRI and CT files (typically stored on CDs). Legally, the doctor's office must provide them. This can be useful if you want to get a second opinion or if your child's case of hip dysplasia is complex. If you are moving, it is a good idea to keep a personal copy of medical records so that you can provide them to the doctor you select in your new location. Some parents have found looking at the medical records helps them clarify their child's condition.

How Doctors Talk about Hip Dysplasia

Each case of hip dysplasia is unique. That said, doctors commonly use certain terms to describe aspects of this condition. Learning these terms will help you understand your child's individual case of hip dysplasia and the treatment that is needed. This section explains terms that you are likely to come across. They are listed in alphabetical order.

● Acetabular Dysplasia

With this form of dysplasia, the hip socket is not the right shape, and it stays that way, which makes the hip unstable. Typically, with hip dysplasia, the hip socket is too shallow. In severe cases, the child's hip might have no hip sockets at all. Conversely, a child who has Down syndrome and hip dysplasia may have hip sockets that are too deep.

● Congenital Dysplasia of the Hip (CDH)

Years ago, all cases of hip dysplasia were called congenital dysplasia of the hip (CDH), and in some countries that is still the case. In the

United States, CDH now describes only cases when a baby is born with hip dysplasia. During the final four weeks before birth, the position of the baby inside the womb can make hip dysplasia more likely, especially if the baby is in a breech or frank breech position. See "Breech Position or Multiples" on page 41 and also "Teratologic Dislocation of the Hip" on page 39.

● Dislocated Hip

With a dislocated hip, the ball at the top of the thighbone (femoral head) is outside the hip socket. The doctor checks to see if it can go into the socket easily. It is important to get the femoral head inside the hip socket so that the hip joint can develop correctly. If the hip joint remains dislocated over a period of time while the child is growing, the joint cannot develop normally. A dislocatable hip is in the right position, but it can be dislocated.

● Ligament Laxity and Flexibility

The hip joint is supported by ligaments and muscles around the hip and pelvis. A ligament is a short band of connective tissue that connects two bones or holds together a joint. Ligament laxity, also called loose ligaments, hypermobility, or double jointed, is common in children who are born with or develop hip dysplasia. It can be hereditary, or it can be present in a baby due to the natural hormones released during pregnancy that relax the mother's ligaments for childbirth. Many babies with ligament laxity outgrow the condition within a couple of months after birth. Doctors take ligament laxity into consideration when creating a treatment plan for hip dysplasia.

Ligament laxity is sometimes confused with flexibility. Flexibility is the ability of muscles to readily adapt to changes in position or alignment. Flexibility allows joints to move through the full range of motion. Flexibility and ligament laxity are different things, but they are related and both affect mobility and stability. For example, if a person has loose ligaments, his or her joints might have excessive movement and therefore lead to longer (and more flexible) muscles. Loose ligaments are less able to stabilize joints than normal (tighter) ligaments. This means the joint can move beyond its normal range of motion. As a result, muscles surrounding the hip have to work harder to maintain stability.

● Leg-Length Discrepancy

A leg-length discrepancy means that one leg is longer than the other. This can happen if one hip is dislocated while a child's bones are growing and developing. If the legs are close to the same length after the hip joint is in the right position, the child might need a shoe insert for the foot of the shorter leg.

Some types of surgery to correct hip dysplasia can result in a leg-length discrepancy. The pediatric orthopedic surgeon does what is possible to minimize this. The doctor might need to do a femoral osteotomy if one leg is a lot longer than the other. A femoral osteotomy is a surgical procedure in which the doctor makes a cut in the thighbone (femur). See "Femoral Osteotomy" on page 112 for more information about this surgery.

● Low Muscle Tone

Some children who have hip dysplasia develop poor muscle tone in the muscles that support the hips. This can happen if the child has an improper stance or from lack of use if he or she cannot crawl or stand normally. This problem is temporary unless a child has other medical conditions such as central core disease or hypotonia, conditions that are both characterized by muscle weakness, in addition to hip dysplasia. You can help your child's muscle tone to improve by encouraging your child to roll, crawl, and walk. Usually physical therapy is not needed for young children with hip dysplasia. If your child needs surgery and a cast, it is normal for the child to have low muscle tone when the cast is removed. See "Regaining Muscle Strength" on page 155.

● Remodeling

In a medical context, remodeling refers to an ongoing, normal process in which new bone gradually grows and old bone tissue is absorbed. This is how doctors and nurses sometimes describe the process of improving the shape of the bones in the pelvis. For example, the doctor might mention pelvic remodeling when talking about how treatment for hip dysplasia encourages a shallow hip socket (acetabulum) to deepen so that the hip is more stable.

● Subluxation

With subluxation, the top of the thighbone (femoral head) is partially in contact with the hip socket. A subluxatable hip is in the right position, but it can partially dislocate.

● Teratologic Dislocation of the Hip

With teratologic dislocation of the hip, one or both hips did not develop properly before the baby was born. The hips are dislocated, and the top of the thighbone cannot be moved into the hip socket. This condition occurs along with other congenital or neurological conditions. The most common are arthrogryposis (multiple joint contractures) and myelomeningocele (a spinal defect).

Babies or children with teratologic dislocation of the hip usually need a hip surgery called an open reduction to move the hips into the right position. Because these cases are more complicated than usual, other problems might need to be treated before the hip dysplasia. For example, in babies with arthrogryposis, hip dysplasia treatment follows any foot or knee surgeries that are needed. Hip dysplasia treatment usually is started before the baby is one year old.

● Toeing In (Femoral Anteversion)

Toeing in or being "pigeon toed" is common for toddlers and occurs twice as often in girls as in boys. With this condition, the thighbone (femur) is twisted inward, causing the knees and toes to point inward. This can make the child look bowlegged. Children often outgrow this without treatment. It also can be caused by stiff hip muscles. If you notice that your child is toeing in, mention it to your child's doctor.

● Toeing Out

Some children with hip dysplasia toe out when the hip is out of position. In some cases, the foot can turn out so far that it is almost pointing backward. Other children toe out when they are learning to walk, even if they do not have hip problems. Shoes with good arch support sometimes help to correct that problem. If you notice that your child is toeing out, this, too, should be mentioned to your child's doctor.

● *Unstable Hip*

The top of the thighbone (femoral head) can come out of the hip socket. Some newborns have unstable hips that resolve within the first few weeks after birth. If the problem continues, it can be associated with hip dysplasia.

If Hip Dysplasia Is Only Part of the Picture

Some medical conditions make hip dysplasia more likely to occur. In the following quote, Patti Streeter describes her daughter Megan's treatments for several medical conditions.

> Our daughter Megan was born in China. She has spina bifida. We adopted her when she was two and a half years old. She had spinal surgery when she was four years old, and foot tendon transfer surgery when she was five years old. Megan had a right hip shelf augmentation [pelvic osteotomy surgery] and a femoral osteotomy. She was seven and a half years old. She spent thirteen weeks in the spica cast. Then she was in a Rhino [hip abduction] brace for six weeks, full-time except for physical therapy and bathing. Then she was allowed to go to six or seven hours out of the brace each day for six weeks. After that, she only needed to use the Rhino brace while sleeping, which she continues to do. She's scheduled to have her hardware [pins from the osteotomy surgery] removed next month.
>
> [Patti]

The following sections describe a number of conditions that can sometimes be associated with hip dysplasia and explain how doctors typically approach treatment of multiple conditions. The treatments are listed in alphabetical order.

● *Arthrogryposis*

Arthrogryposis, also known as arthrogryposis multiplex congenita (AMC), is a condition in which there are multiple joint contractures throughout the body that are present at birth. (A muscle contracture means that the muscle has shortened and cannot easily stretch.) Any foot and knee surgeries that are needed are done first, followed by treatment for hip problems. Some types of bilateral (both sides) hip dislocations can be treated with stretching and soft-tissue releases; others require a surgical procedure called a reduction. A unilateral (only one side) hip dislocation usually requires a reduction. Hip surgery is recommended before the baby is one year old. See "Reduction" on page 100 and Chapter 6, "If Your Child Needs Surgery," beginning on page 78.

● *Breech Position or Multiples*

Babies who are carried in a breech position or are multiples such as twins or triplets are more likely to have hip dysplasia and other conditions related to their position in the womb. For example, a breech baby might have a foot that turns inward or a skull that is asymmetrical. If this is the case, it is usually noticeable at birth and is evaluated by the doctor. Because breech babies are at increased risk for hip dysplasia, the American Academy of Pediatrics (AAP) recommends hip ultrasounds for them even if the hips seem fine when the doctor examines them. The breech position is not associated with the same problems that occur in teratologic hip dysplasia.

● *Bowlegs*

Bowlegs in babies are considered normal before the age of 18 months due to the position of a baby's legs before birth. Bowlegs are more common in situations when space in the womb was limited such as for a breech, firstborn, or large baby—the same factors that increase the risk of hip dysplasia. As long as the baby gets enough vitamin D and his or her milestones for sitting, crawling, and standing are normal, observation is all that is needed until the age of eighteen to twenty-four months. Vitamin D is important for bones to grow strong and straight. Your child's pediatrician can provide information about how much vitamin D your child needs. Bowlegs usually resolve after a child starts walking.

● Central Core Disease

Central core disease is a neurological disorder that is usually inherited. People with this rare disorder have muscle cells that contain cores. If a doctor believes a child might have central core disease, a muscle biopsy is taken and sent to a laboratory to confirm the diagnosis. Typically, people with this disorder have weakness in their legs, but other muscle groups also can be affected. Hip dislocations are common due to the lack of muscular development in the hip area. Scoliosis (a curved spine), and problems with the foot and knee might also be present. If a child's hip dislocates, the pediatric orthopedic doctor needs to know that the child has central core disease, as the child might have more trouble tolerating anesthesia if surgery is required.

● Cerebral Palsy

Cerebral palsy (CP) is a developmental disability that causes uncontrollable movement and posture. Symptoms typically appear within the first few years of life and do not get progressively worse over time. CP is not caused by problems with muscles or nerves. The motor areas in the brain are damaged or do not develop correctly. Some children with CP also have other neurological problems such as epilepsy, mental impairments, growth problems, and vision or hearing problems.

There is a wide range of symptoms among individuals who have CP. Children with mild cases have difficulty with fine motor coordination and might move somewhat awkwardly. In other cases, all limbs are severely affected.

A child with CP who also has hip dysplasia needs to have an individual treatment plan for managing the CP and treating the hip dysplasia. Depending on the severity of the case, the hip dysplasia might need to be treated to prevent problems with pain either in childhood or in later life. For example, the child might find sitting painful. If surgery is needed, it is done before age four, if possible, to encourage normal hip-joint development and because it is easier for a parent to move and care for a younger child.

Connective Tissue Disorders

Most people with hip dysplasia do not have connective tissue disorders. However, some people with connective tissue disorders are prone to hip dysplasia and dislocated joints. This is due to problems with the soft tissue that connect the joints. This type of hip dysplasia can be harder to treat than others. Typically treatment for hip dysplasia is the same with a connective tissue disorder. The child is checked for other problems and treated for them as well. Connective tissue disorders that are associated with hip dysplasia include the following.

Brittle Bone Disorder (Osteogenesis Imperfecta)

In this disorder, Type 1 collagen is not produced normally, leading to bones that break easily. Collagen is a strong, fibrous protein in connective tissues and bones. A skin biopsy or genetic test might be run to diagnose this syndrome.

Ehlers-Danlos syndrome (EDS)

People with Ehlers-Danlos syndrome (EDS) have a defect in their collagen and often have unstable joints. A skin biopsy is used to test for EDS, which runs in families. People who test positive for EDS Type VII typically have dislocated hips.

Larsen Syndrome

The condition known as Larsen syndrome often results in malformed joints. A geneticist might order a skeletal survey. This is a series of X rays taken to examine the child's bone and joint structure.

Clubfoot (Talipes)

Clubfoot, also called Talipes equinovarus or Talipes, is a disorder in which the foot is turned downward and inward at birth and remains in this position. Clubfoot is treated as early as possible. If a child has both hip dysplasia and clubfoot, usually the doctor treats the clubfoot first and then treats the hip dysplasia. It is rare for a child to have both clubfoot and hip dysplasia.

● Down Syndrome

Down syndrome is a chromosomal disorder in which all or part of an extra 21st chromosome is present. Down syndrome has several associated conditions, which can include hip dysplasia or other hip problems that do not surface until adulthood. With Down syndrome, the hip sockets typically are deeper than usual, which is different from most other types of hip dysplasia in which the sockets are too shallow. See "Osteotomy Surgery" on page 105 and "Considerations for Children with Down Syndrome" on page 110.

● Head Shape (Positional Plagiocelphaly)

A baby's skull can become flattened after birth if the child is always placed in the same position on his back. This is called positional plagiocelphaly. To make this less likely to occur, give your baby interesting things to look at in a variety of directions. For example, babies often look at the bedroom door. If you alternate which end of the crib you put your baby's head, then he will sometimes be looking to his right, and other times be looking to the left. This makes it less likely that the back of his head will become flat. Some babies wear helmets to correct a problem with head shape. This can be done at the same time as treatment for hip dysplasia.

● Impingement

Impingement, also called femoroacetabular impingement (FAI) is a condition in which the shape of the bones in the hip joint causes pain or a pinching sensation in certain positions. FAI is not caused by hip dysplasia, but the two conditions can occur together. FAI is treated either with arthroscopy or hip surgery.

● Tethered Spinal Cord

A tethered spinal cord can also be called a neural tube defect or "closed" spina bifida. Some babies have been identified as having a neurogenic problem that includes a tethered spinal cord, clubfoot, and hip dysplasia. The neurosurgery department and the pediatric orthopedic department work together to develop a course of treatment for these conditions. A pediatric neurosurgeon must correct the problem with the spinal cord first. Usually the clubfoot is treated next, followed by the hip dysplasia.

● Torticollis

A newborn with this condition has limited motion on one side of the neck. The baby might always look in the same direction, and the head could be tilted. In many cases, this can be corrected with gentle stretching exercises done by a parent or physical therapist. You can encourage your child to look in different directions by putting toys or a mirror on the side where you want her to look. Even if she looks only for a short time, this can help. The doctor might give you a referral to meet with a physical therapist. In some cases, surgery is needed to release the tight muscle. Treatment is important so that the child will have a full range of motion. Untreated, the child could always have limited motion of the neck. The torticollis and hip dysplasia can be treated at the same time.

Health-Care Workers:
Who Does What?

During treatment you will come in contact with health-care professionals. This section explains the training and role of health-care workers who might be involved in your child's care. Treatment plans vary, so you might not meet with each type of health-care worker that is described in this section.

● Anesthesiologist or Pediatric Anesthesiologist

Anesthetics are drugs that prevent or reduce pain. An anesthesiologist is a doctor who completed an internship and residency in anesthesiology and is certified by the American Board of Anesthesiologists. A pediatric anesthesiologist has additional training in using anesthetics for babies and children.

● Child Life Specialist

A child life specialist is a health-care professional who helps children and their families cope with procedures and issues that come up in a health-care setting such as a hospital. A child life specialist has a bachelor's degree or an advanced degree in a related field and might also be certified.

● Geneticist

A geneticist is a doctor who has studied genetics and is certified by the American Board of Medical Genetics. A pediatric geneticist also completes a residency in pediatrics and is certified by the American Board of Pediatrics. If your child's hip dysplasia could be due to a genetic condition such as Larsen syndrome, you might see a geneticist.

● Nurse Practitioner

A nurse practitioner (NP) is a registered nurse with at least a master's degree, specialized training, and certifications to perform health examinations and prescribe medications. Pediatric NPs specialize in the care of children.

● Orthotist

An orthotist makes and fits orthopedic harnesses and braces prescribed by doctors. Sometimes the orthotist is part of the pediatric orthopedic practice. In other cases, the orthotist has an independent practice or works in an orthotics store.

● Pediatric Orthopedic Surgeon

A pediatric orthopedic surgeon is a doctor who specializes in bone and joint problems in babies and children. This doctor completed an orthopedic surgery residency and also completed additional training in pediatric orthopedics.

● Pediatrician

A pediatrician specializes in treating children. Most pediatricians are members of professional organizations such as the American Academy of Pediatrics.

● Physical Therapist

A physical therapist is trained to work with people of all ages to prevent the onset, or reduce the progression, of conditions resulting from disease, injury, or other causes.

Physician's Assistant

A physician's assistant (PA) is a licensed health-care professional who provides health-care services under the supervision of doctors. In some states, PAs may prescribe some medications.

Radiologist

A radiologist is trained to interpret X rays and to understand how they affect the human body. Some diagnostic radiologists are also trained in ultrasound and MRI.

Health Insurance and Financial Assistance

Whether or not your child has health insurance, spend some time finding out what expenses will be involved in your child's treatment. Some tips for dealing with health insurance and support organizations are provided in this section. Contact information for these organizations is located in the "Resources" chapter.

Some medical expenses might be tax deductible. Tax laws vary from year to year and depend on your individual circumstances. If you must travel a lot for your child's treatment, check with your tax preparer or the appropriate government tax agencies to see if the travel costs, meals, and mileage are tax deductible.

Air and Ground Transportation

If you need to travel for your child's treatment, organizations exist that might be able to help. Air Care Alliance, the National Patient Travel Center, and Angel Flight provide free or reduced-cost transportation for patients in the United States.

Easter Seals

Easter Seals is a nonprofit organization that offers services to caregivers, including support and financial assistance. Some Easter Seals offices have a list of pediatric orthopedic doctors. They can sometimes get a car seat to fit a child in a cast. Easter Seals has many offices throughout the United States.

● Early Intervention Services

The Federal Individuals with Disabilities Education Act requires states to provide early intervention services to children who have been assessed for developmental delays and determined to be eligible. A child with hip dysplasia usually does not qualify for these services. However, these programs can help children who have medical challenges or developmental delays in addition to hip dysplasia. For example, a child with both cerebral palsy and hip dysplasia might qualify for physical therapy. Each state has a separate organization, so you need to contact the one for your location. Most states have programs specifically geared toward children between birth and three years of age.

● Health Insurance

When working with insurance companies, it is important to understand your policy, to stay organized, and to keep records. If your child's case is mild and treatment is straightforward, this could be a simple process. For more complicated cases, you might find that paperwork gets lost, something was not filed correctly, the wrong amount was paid, or nothing was paid for a procedure or item that is covered by your policy. As aggravating as this is, stay calm if you can, and contact the insurance company in a timely manner to correct the problem.

Keep your own records of dates, authorization numbers, and copies of referrals. If you need to call the insurance company, ask for a supervisor or manager. Write down the name and phone number in case of future calls. If the insurance company still refuses to cover a necessary item for your child's treatment, such as a brace, then you can appeal. Ask for a case manager and find out what the appeals process is. If you are struggling with an insurance company, try asking for help from the pediatric orthopedic doctor's office, or the hospital where your child was treated. Either group might be willing to contact the insurance company about the item or procedure in question.

● Ronald McDonald House Charities

The Ronald McDonald House Charities provide a number of services for children. The most well-known of these are the Ronald Mc-

Donald Houses. These houses are located near children's hospitals in a number of cities and towns. Families with children in treatment can stay at a Ronald McDonald House at a reduced rate. In many cases, help is available with meals and transportation to and from the hospital while you are staying at a Ronald McDonald House. Each house has guidelines for guests such as for cleaning the room or suite in which they are staying. For more detailed information, contact the Ronald McDonald House located nearest your destination.

● Shriners Hospitals for Children

Shriners Hospitals for Children are associated with the Shriners organization. These hospitals do not charge for treatment. If your child has health insurance, they cover the portion of the treatment costs that your insurance does not. If your child has poor health insurance, or no health insurance, they will still accept the child for treatment. Shriners will provide a second opinion, even if you do not choose to use them for treatment. If you do not live near a Shriners hospital, the Shriners organization is often able to arrange transportation.

● Texas Scottish Rite Children's Hospital

Texas Scottish Rite Hospital for Children provides orthopedic treatment for Texas children, regardless of the ability to pay. This hospital was founded by the Masons and is not associated with Shriners Hospitals for Children.

Family and Medical Leave Act

In the United States, depending on the size of the company for which you work, the Family Medical Leave Act (FMLA) might allow you to take up to 12 weeks of unpaid leave per year to care for a family member. This is the same act that covers maternity leave. If your child needs surgery and you can afford to take the time off, this can be helpful while he or she is recovering.

Child Care

If your child goes to child care, talk to the provider about your child's treatment. If your child is wearing a Pavlik harness or brace, make sure that the provider understands how long it must be worn. For a cast, explain how important it is to keep the cast clean and dry.

Show the child care provider how to change diapers or to assist with toileting depending on the age of your child. If you have items that work well at home such as a beanbag chair or stroller, get a duplicate set if you can. Bring the extra set to the child-care provider so that he or she will be set up to succeed with your child. If your child is mobile, the provider needs to know. Stay the first time or two that you bring your child to the child-care location. That will give the child-care provider time to learn how to care for your child and to ask any questions that come up.

If your child needs surgery and you want to take time off work to handle his or her care yourself, check to see if you are eligible for up to 12 weeks of unpaid leave through the Family Medical Leave Act (FMLA).

Brothers and Sisters

Take the time to talk to all of the children in the family about their sibling's treatment. Often, older siblings have questions about why treatment is needed. Explain that the treatment may take a long time, but it will help the child to avoid having problems later.

> What I found helped my four-year-old when his younger sister was diagnosed, was to put him in charge of getting Claudia her toys. He loved it that he was in charge of helping her to get better.
>
> **[NANCY]**

Sometimes siblings worry about the child in treatment, especially when the patient is fussy. The sibling might feel bad and even cry. Other children might be jealous of the extra attention that a child needs while in treatment. Let all of your children know that you love everyone in the family just the same.

Brothers and sisters can be a big help when one child is in a cast. They can bring toys to the child, or pick up his or her dropped toys

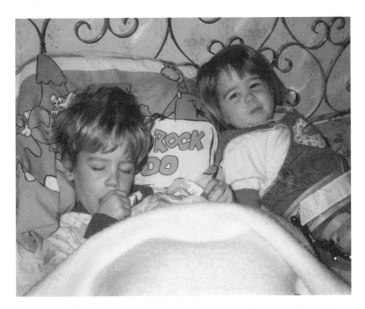

FIGURE 19. Claudia, wearing a brace, is shown with her brother Kyle.
(Photo courtesy of Nancy Sanders)

and other items. Some families let older children decorate a sibling patient's plaster cast by drawing or coloring on it. Some children enjoy reading books to or playing with a laid up brother or sister. (Your children might especially enjoy a children's book such as *When Molly Was in the Hospital: A Book for Brothers and Sisters of Hospitalized Children* by Debbie Duncan.) The important thing is to have fun together when you can and keep a positive attitude. If people make comments about the "poor little baby," tell them that your child is doing well. Brothers and sisters will take their cues from you.

Hip dysplasia is common enough that pediatric orthopedic doctors know how to treat it. At the same time, it is uncommon enough that most people have never heard of it unless they know someone with the condition. The doctor can explain medical treatment, but treating hip dysplasia involves treating the hips—which means that caring for a child who is in treatment affects many aspects of family life. The next chapters in this book offer practical advice from parents with experience caring for babies with hip dysplasia.

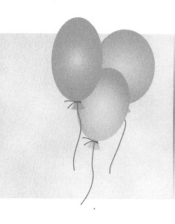

4

Treatment with a Pavlik Harness

If hip dysplasia is caught early, the Pavlik harness is an effective treatment over 90 percent of the time. The Pavlik harness is the first line of treatment for almost all babies up to the age of six months. It can work for older infants, but the success rate decreases with age. Some doctors have had success with babies up to ten months old with some adjustments based on the baby's size and age. A consideration for older babies is that after wearing the Pavlik harness for four weeks, if an ultrasound or an arthrogram (X ray with dye) shows that the Pavlik harness is not working, the baby should stop wearing it. If the Pavlik harness is working for an older baby, after two or three months, the baby typically starts wearing a hip abduction brace instead.

Note: If a child is too old for a Pavlik harness, the doctor will recommend a hip abduction brace or surgery. For more information about these treatments, see Chapter 5, "Treatment with a Brace (Hip Abduction Orthosis)," beginning on page 65 and Chapter 6, "If Your Child Needs Surgery," beginning on page 78.

The Pavlik harness works by keeping the baby's legs apart and at the ideal angle in the hip sockets to encourage better hip development. Treatment in the Pavlik harness is often tried for six weeks. If it is working well, it can be continued until the baby is six months old. Figure 20 shows a baby wearing a Pavlik harness.

The pediatric orthopedic doctor decides whether to prescribe the Pavlik harness based on the age of the baby and the results of the hip exam and ultrasound. In making a decision about the harness, the doctor takes the following into consideration:

FIGURE 20. A baby wearing a Pavlik harness. *(Photo courtesy of Rhino Pediatric Orthopedic Designs, Inc.)*

* If a newborn baby's hips are unstable, some doctors wait until the baby is six to eight weeks of age to see if the hips stabilize without treatment. Unstable hips are common among newborns.

* A positive Ortolani test (see "The Ortolani Test for Newborns" on page 15) identifies a dislocated hip in which the thighbone can go back into the hip socket. A Pavlik harness usually works, but in some cases other treatment is needed.

* A positive Barlow's test (see "The Barlow's Test" on page 16) identifies an unstable hip that could benefit from the Pavlik harness to keep it from dislocating.

In the following situations, the Pavlik harness is not recommended because it will not help the baby's hips:

* A baby who is older than six months of age is too big and strong for the Pavlik harness to work. At this age, a baby will either wear a brace or need surgery.

* A baby born with teratologic hip dysplasia needs surgery to correct the problem.

* If something prevents the ball at the top of the thighbone (femoral head) from fitting inside the hip socket normally, surgery is needed. In some cases, fatty tissue called pulvinar has collected inside the hip socket and must be removed; in other cases a tendon or other connective tissue is blocking the hip socket.

❋ A premature baby might be too small to wear a harness. If this is the case, the doctor will prescribe treatment when the child is a little bigger.

Understanding Treatment

When the pediatric orthopedic doctor fits your baby with the Pavlik harness, make sure that you understand the treatment. Some questions that you might want to ask are listed here:

❋ Can the harness be removed? The answer to this question depends on your baby's individual case of hip dysplasia and can change over time as your baby's hips improve. Especially in the beginning of treatment, the doctor might feel strongly that it is important for your baby to wear the harness 24 hours a day. If this is the case, removing the harness at home reduces its effectiveness. It could take your baby's hips longer to get better.

❋ What kind of clothes can my baby wear under the harness?

❋ Who will adjust the harness?

❋ Should I call this office if I have a question or problem with the way the harness fits?

❋ How often should I bring the baby in to be checked?

Fitting or Adjusting a Pavlik Harness

The doctor puts the Pavlik harness on the baby and adjusts the straps to get the hip joints in the correct position for healthy development.

Doctors typically follow these steps to put on a Pavlik harness:

1. First the halter is put on, allowing enough room to put a hand between the baby's chest and the harness.

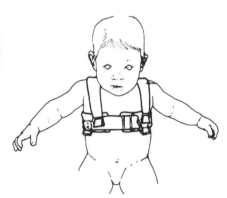

FIGURE 21. The chest strap is fastened first.

The chest strap of the halter is worn about ½ inch (1 cm) below the armpits (see Figure 21). This strap supports the straps to the stirrups, keeping the baby's knees at a 90-degree angle. The chest strap is adjusted as the baby grows but can change as little as 1 inch (2.5 cm) during ten weeks of treatment.

2. The baby's feet are put into the stirrups one at a time (see Figure 22).

3. The doctor connects the straps from the halter to the stirrups and adjusts the lengths as necessary (see Figure 23).

4. The doctor connects the back straps and adjusts the length (see Figure 24).

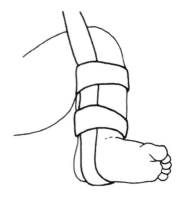

For a link to an online video that demonstrates putting on and removing the Pavlik harness ("Pavlik Harness Application Part 1 and Part 2"), see "IHDI Online" in the "Online Video Resources" section on page 190.

Only the doctor should adjust the back straps. The back straps keep the

FIGURE 22. The foot strap is fastened.

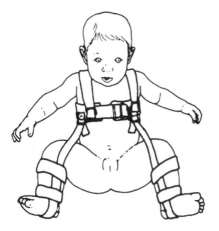

FIGURE 23. The chest strap and feet straps are in place.

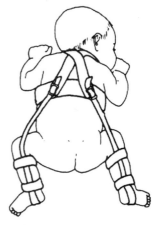

FIGURE 24. A baby, in a correctly fitted Pavlik harness, shown from behind.
(Illustrations courtesy of the Journal of Bone & Joint Surgery)

baby's legs in the frog-leg position and prevent the baby's legs from coming together in front of his or her body. The legs should be at least fist-width apart, which is about 3½ inches (9 cm).

While the harness is worn, the doctor checks to make sure the hips are stable and not dislocated to encourage healthy hip development. Some doctors mark the straps in case the harness has to be removed to make sure that it is put back on in the correct position. The doctor might also give you an instruction sheet that explains the steps involved in putting on the harness.

The doctor will show you how to lift the baby while he or she is wearing the harness and how to lay down the baby. While the baby is wearing the Pavlik harness, he or she should not take a bath. You can give your baby sponge baths between checkups. Ask the doctor if you can take your baby out of the harness an hour before you come in for a checkup so that you can give him or her a bath on that day.

As the child grows, the Pavlik harness is adjusted. Usually parents can adjust the chest strap if it gets too tight between doctor visits. All other adjustments are made at the doctor's office during visits either every two weeks or every week, depending on the doctor and on how fast the baby is growing.

Femoral Nerve Palsy, a Rare Complication

Femoral nerve palsy occurs in about 2 to 3 percent of babies who wear the Pavlik harness, typically within the first week of wear. Femoral nerve palsy has an effect similar to when someone's leg "falls asleep" when it has been in the same position for an extended time. If this happens, the baby is not in pain, but because the femoral nerve controls the leg muscle, the baby cannot straighten his or her leg (see Figure 25). This condition nearly always resolves with a change in position.

Doctors check for femoral nerve palsy during treatment with the Pavlik harness. If it occurs, either the baby stops wearing the harness, or the angle of the harness is changed. Femoral nerve palsy is more common in older, heavier babies whose hip dysplasia is more serious, such as a baby with a stiff, dislocated hip.

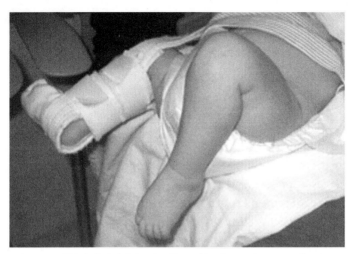

FIGURE 25. This baby's left leg is affected by femoral nerve palsy.

Pavlik Harness at Home

The first week with the harness is the hardest. Expect your baby to be fussy as he or she adjusts to wearing it. Your child might be clingy, and it will most likely take him or her a while to adjust to new sleeping positions. If a baby has just learned how to roll over, he or she might be frustrated while figuring out how to roll over while wearing the harness. Hang in there. Your baby needs this treatment. Bear in mind that babies are resilient and can adapt. You can too. You will work out a new routine, and you will get better at it with practice.

If you are breast-feeding your baby, you can continue to do so while your baby wears the Pavlik harness. You can try laying the baby sideways across your chest while he or she is supported on a bed pillow, or the football hold might work for you. To use the football hold, place your baby's feet under your arm with his face toward your breast, and use your arm to hold your baby like a football.

Most everyday products for babies except for long pants work fine for a baby in a Pavlik harness. You might need to make some adjustments such as buying large socks. You probably can use the same infant carrier, car seat, and stroller (umbrella strollers usually work well). While your baby is wearing the harness, his or her legs go out to the side.

Tip: If your car seat doesn't work, look for a car seat with low sides. Go to a store with a large selection and try your baby in different seats to see which one works best for him or her. For more information, see "Car Seats—You Might Need a New One" on page 72.

● Diapering

For a baby wearing a harness, many parents find disposable diapers easier to manage than cloth. When cloth diapers are wet, the urine can wick into the straps of the harness. For either disposable or cloth diapers, you can use a piece of cloth to keep the leg straps of the harness away from the mess. Lift the baby up under the thighs, not by the legs. The diaper always needs to go under the harness.

● Skin Care

Skin irritation is common in children who wear a harness. Some places to check are in the creases of the child's thighs and behind the knees. If the skin is irritated, clean it gently with a soft washcloth and apply a diaper cream such as Balmex or Neosporin. Aquaphor Healing Ointment also helps keep the skin healthy.

● Lining the Straps

Some children get minor skin irritation at the neck from the harness straps. You can tuck fleece around the shoulder strap to stop the problem. Fleece is sold at fabric stores, but you do not need to sew to use it. Cut a square and tuck it around the strap. If it gets dirty, wash it with the baby's laundry. Another option is to take little socks, cut out the toes, and thread the shoulder straps through.

If you like to sew, you can make a lining to cover the harness straps. Sew a simple tube from silky fabric to go over the strap. You can shift the lining up out of the way when adjusting the straps. You can also use silk on the chest strap and moleskin on the hard plastic parts of the harness. Putting moleskin on the straps does not work well because it can harden if it gets wet.

● Clothing Tips

To change your baby's shirt, remove the harness shoulder straps, one side at a time. You can change your baby's socks by removing the bottom foot straps. Some suggestions about clothes for babies in the Pavlik harness are listed here:

* Avoid pants or pull-up diaper covers because they might not fit over the harness.

* For shirts, try pullover and kimono styles.

* For onesies, you can use Add-a-Size garment extenders available through One Step Ahead. These make leg openings bigger so that they do not press on the harness straps.

* For dresses, use the next size up.

* Use toddler-size socks to fit over the harness.

* When the baby sleeps, use a T-shirt and a sleep sack in a larger size to fit over the legs, or cut the bottom out of a sleep sack.

* If you like to sew, you can make diaper covers that open at the sides. Patterns can be bought at fabric stores.

One mother from the Hip-baby online support group (www.hip -baby.org) was happy to discover socks that look like dressy tights and shoes for her daughter.

My four-month-old daughter, Grace, has been in a Pavlik since day four. As the holidays approached, our friends and families gave us beautiful little dresses and tights for her. I was discouraged because the tights were not working out. I found a company called Trumpette (sold on various websites), which makes baby socks. They are adorable and fit nicely over her harness. We skipped the tights, but it looked as if Grace was wearing them because of the socks. They wash and dry very well, and I always receive compliments when she is wearing them!   **[HIP-BABY DISCUSSION GROUP]**

Removing a Pavlik Harness

Each baby's treatment is planned by the pediatric orthopedic doctor. One baby must wear a harness 24 hours a day, while another needs to wear it only for part of the day or at night. In many cases, a baby starts out wearing the harness 24 hours a day. As the hips improve, the doctor lets the parents take it off for part of the day. If the harness can be removed, the doctor's marks showing you where the straps go will be especially helpful so that you can see how to put it back on the baby. If your baby becomes ill during the time he or she is wearing the harness, the doctor might allow you to remove it. In this case, do not unfasten the shoulder straps, which are set to keep the baby's legs at the ideal angle. Instead, unfasten the chest and leg straps. If your doctor gave you an instruction sheet when your baby was fitted for the harness, use it as a reference. See "Online Video Resources" on page 189, which includes a link to a video that shows a mother putting a Pavlik harness on her son.

If your baby wears the harness all the time, he or she should not take a bath. You can rely on sponge baths between checkups.

If your doctor allows your child time during the day without a harness, then he or she can ride in a car seat without it. Be sure to keep track of how long the child spends in the car seat so that the time does not exceed the amount of "free time" that is allowed. If your child rides in the car while wearing a Pavlik harness, car seats with low sides usually work the best.

When your baby has been wearing a harness and has had only sponge baths for a long time, you will probably be eager to bathe him or her. From the baby's point of view, however, a bath might seem like a brand new experience. Some babies like baths and happily take to them again. Others scream. If your baby does not like the bath, try sitting in the tub and holding him, or putting a baby chair into the tub to support him. Let your child get used to the water a little at a time. If the weather is good, he or she might like to play in a kiddie pool. For helpful information about bathing your baby, you can ask other parents or try parenting books and magazines.

Cleaning a Pavlik Harness

Cleaning the harness depends on the brand. With some, you can sponge off a mess if you need to. Other harnesses, such as the Rhino Kicker Pavlik harness, can go into the washing machine and dryer. Others are not designed for this, so even using the delicate cycle in a washing machine can make the harness "fuzzy." It can take an hour or two to air dry a harness (especially the part that goes on the baby's back).

One mother offers the following method to wash a harness by hand:

[The harness] was just filthy, and I tried all sorts of things. Finally, I found a great combination of cleaning tips. First, spray the harness with Oxyclean baby spray and let it sit. Scrub and wipe it off. Then, spray on Spray and Wash foam and let it sit again. Fill up a bucket with really hot water, putting in the detergent as it fills. Soak the harness for 20 minutes. Rinse, wring it out, and let it sit out in the sun to help bleach it a bit. Let it dry in the dryer for the last little bit. It takes about an hour (as long as he is allowed to be out of the harness). I also cut off the little fuzzies that appear on the felt part of the harness. I do it every Saturday, and it's HORRIBLE by the next Saturday. This works great for us!   **[HIP-BABY DISCUSSION GROUP]**

This mother clearly has a knack for figuring out how to get things really clean and was able to develop a system that worked for her. These instructions might be helpful if you find yourself hand washing a dirty or soiled Pavlik harness. Depending on your circumstances (and the state of the harness), you could try some or all of her suggestions or come up with your own ideas.

Another idea: Some families have purchased a spare harness, but the feasibility of this depends on the cost, and that varies according to where you live. For example, a mother in Ecuador may pay $18 for her baby's harness, but a similar harness can cost up to $165 in the United States.

Comforting a Fussy Baby

It can be hard to tell if a baby is being fussy because of a problem with the harness or due to another cause such as teething, a virus, or a common ailment such as an ear infection. How a baby reacts to wearing the harness can be influenced by temperament and her age. For example, a three-month old baby who is used to life without the harness will need a period of adjustment to get used to new sleeping positions and the sensation of wearing the harness. A newborn fitted with a harness will have a different experience. Here are some suggestions to soothe a fussy baby:

* Try a diaper change. Check for any skin irritation or diaper rash.

* Check the leg creases. If the skin is irritated, apply a barrier cream such as Balmex or Neosporin.

* Consider the same ideas you would if your baby was not in the harness. Your baby might enjoy a different position or be hungry, need to burp, or want to be held.

If you are worried that the harness does not fit correctly or you think your child is in pain, consult your doctor's office.

Sleeping

The first night spent in a harness is typically the hardest for a baby, but it can take a week or so for some babies to adjust to sleeping well while wearing it. Below are some suggestions to help to ease the adjustment period.

* Prop up your baby's legs. Use a rolled-up blanket or cushion under the baby's legs, especially if one is dangling. As the leg muscles stretch, you can reduce the height of the props until your child doesn't need them anymore.

* Consider using a swing. If your baby can't sleep in the crib, he or she might be able to sleep in a swing.

* Try tummy time. Laying your baby on his stomach helps stretch out muscles, even if it is for a very short time during the day. If your baby doesn't like to be on his tummy, try letting him lie on top of you.

* Check if your baby could be teething or have other problems. If your child is inconsolable, maybe the problem is not the harness. Check the same things you would otherwise look for in a fussy baby: teething, an ear infection, or symptoms of other ailments.

Contact your doctor if you are worried about your child or believe he or she is in pain. The Pavlik harness should not be painful. Checking with the doctor can help you figure out what is causing the problem. For information about pain relief, see "Pain Management at Home" on page 97.

Checkups for a Baby in a Pavlik Harness

During treatment with the Pavlik harness, the pediatric orthopedic doctor schedules visits to see how everything is going. How often the doctor sees the baby depends on his or her individual treatment plan. The following quote illustrates how one baby's hip progressed while she was wearing a Pavlik harness.

> [Zoey's] hip is in place now, and she'll only have to wear the Pavlik for six to eight more weeks. I consider that excellent news! Her hip socket was shallow, so her hip could come out of place. Now, there is cartilage that has formed, which will turn into bone. Then the ball joint will rub that new bone down and make the socket deeper. Interesting how that works! She will only be around six months old when she is able to get it off, if everything goes well. We only have to go to the doctor every two to three weeks now instead of every week. **[CATIE]**

The doctor examines the baby's hips, and usually has X rays taken while the baby is in the harness. Ultrasound or MRI might be used if the baby's bones are not yet solid enough to show up on X rays. Some doctors discuss the AI (acetabular index) and percent coverage for the hip sockets. For more information about these topics see "Interpreting X Rays" on page 23. If the hips are improving, treatment in the Pavlik harness continues, and the doctor will schedule the next appointment for your baby.

Babies can roll and learn to sit up while wearing the Pavlik harness. However, there is a wide range of what is normal. If your baby does not roll over or sit while wearing the Pavlik harness, try not to worry about it. Talk to your child's doctor about any concerns that you have in this area. Babies with other medical challenges, such as cerebral palsy, can have developmental delays not related to hip dysplasia.

When Treatment with the Pavlik Harness Ends

Many babies are finished with treatment after the Pavlik harness is removed and then need only follow-up checkups. Your pediatric orthopedic doctor will tell you how often your child's hips should be checked as he or she grows and develops. Other babies will then wear a brace (hip abduction orthosis) or need surgery. For more information about these treatments, see Chapter 5, "Treatment with a Brace (Hip Abduction Orthosis)," on page 65 and Chapter 6, "If Your Child Needs Surgery," on page 78.

If your baby is finished with treatment, congratulations! Your baby might be uncomfortable for a short time as he or she adjusts to life without the harness. Many babies start kicking very soon. The baby's legs might take a day or so to come down from the frog-leg position. If your child has other conditions besides hip dysplasia that make it hard for him or her to move the legs, discuss this with your child's doctor. It can take parents a day or two to adjust as well. As one mother wrote, when her daughter was finished wearing the Pavlik harness:

> It seems so weird to hold her now. We can't remember how to cuddle her in our arms—I'm serious. And her legs...they are SO long. I can't believe how much she has grown since she's had [the harness] on. She almost looks odd in clothes now. We feel like we may break her when we hold her. It will take some getting used to!
>
> **[SUZANNE]**

After successful Pavlik harness treatment when the X ray is normal, the hip has about a 99 percent to continue growing normally. But a small risk remains that the hip socket (acetabulum) could become shallow as the child grows. For this reason, most doctors still recommend X rays at an older age just to catch any shallow sockets.

5

Treatment with a Brace (Hip Abduction Orthosis)

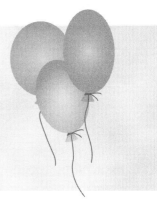

In some cases, a baby or child wears a brace as treatment for hip dysplasia. This chapter describes treatment with a brace and offers tips for caring for a baby or child who is wearing a brace. The kind of brace used to treat hip dysplasia is called a hip abduction orthosis. These braces come in many different styles and are made of a variety of materials.

Generally, brace treatment begins before the baby is six months of age. However, in some instances it may be helpful to begin brace wear in a baby up to one year of age, or in older children after a cast has been removed. Research is in progress regarding the Hoffman-Daimler method, which uses bracing up to two and a half years of age.

The brace works by keeping the child's legs apart and at the best angle to encourage the hips to develop correctly. The pediatric orthopedic doctor prescribes the brace but usually does not fit the child with the brace. Most likely you will take your child to an orthotist. An orthotist is trained to design and fit braces that are prescribed by doctors.

Some examples of situations in which a doctor might prescribe a brace are listed here:

* The doctor believes a brace would be more effective for the baby than the Pavlik harness. A brace might work even if the Pavlik harness did not.

* The brace is a follow-up treatment after a child finishes treatment with a cast. The brace is often worn for the same length of time as the cast. For example, if the cast was worn for 12 weeks, then the brace is worn for 12 weeks. At first the brace is worn full-time. As the hips get better, the doctor often will let the brace be removed for part of the day.

Doctors typically do not prescribe a brace to treat hip dysplasia in the following circumstances:

* If the baby is over six months old when diagnosed with hip dysplasia.

* When a child is old enough to remove a brace, it might be discontinued or used only at night.

* If the ball at the top of the thighbone (femoral head) cannot go into the hip socket, then a brace is not effective. If this is the case, surgery is needed. See Chapter 6, "If Your Child Needs Surgery," on page 78.

Understanding the Brace

When the pediatric orthopedic doctor prescribes the brace, ask any questions that you have to make sure that you understand the treatment. Some questions that you might want to ask are listed here:

* How long can my child be out of the brace each day?

* Can I remove the brace for diaper changes or for toileting?

* How often and for how long can I remove the brace to bathe my child?

* Can clothing be worn under the brace?

Many kinds of braces are used to treat hip dysplasia. They are made of plastics, steel, leather, or a combination of these materials. Most come in several sizes. Some braces, such as the Scottish Rite brace, are called walking abduction braces. They are heavier than the other braces, but they make it easier for the child to walk because there is a hinge at the top. The doctor selects the brace that is best for the baby or child. Some braces are described in the following sections. They are listed in alphabetical order.

◉ Basko B-Hip Abduction Orthosis

This brace is made of soft plastic and is worn on top of clothing.

It is used for young babies who are not yet walking. The brace should fit comfortably on your baby. You should be able to insert one finger between the leg cuff and your baby's thigh, or four fingers between the abdominal strap and your baby's body.

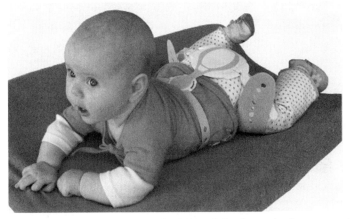

FIGURE 26. A baby wearing a Basko B-Hip abduction orthosis *(Photo courtesy of Fillauer, LLC)*

Note that Fillauer provides detailed instructions for putting on this brace. See the caregiver instructions in the pdf document "Basko B-Hip CDH Hip Abduction Orthosis," available at www.fillauer.com.

◉ Correctio Brace

This brace can be worn on top of clothing. It is more commonly used in Australia and Europe than in the United States.

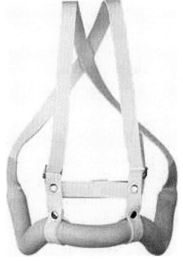

FIGURE 27. A Correctio brace *(Photo courtesy of Teufel International)*

● Denis Brown Abduction Splint

This brace has a strip of padded aluminum around the back. Two rings go around the legs, and cloth straps go over the shoulders (see Figure 28).

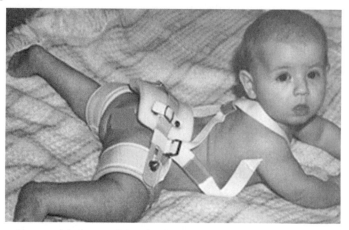

FIGURE 28. A baby wearing a Denis Brown abduction splint *(Photo courtesy of Steps Charity)*

Your doctor might prescribe a Denis Brown abduction splint after a Pavlik harness or spica cast is removed. You can hand wash this brace with warm water and use a towel to dry it. Your baby can wear clothing made of thin cotton material under the brace to minimize skin irritation from sweat. Your orthotist might be able to provide fabric for this purpose. Do not use oils or lotions on your baby's skin while he or she is wearing this brace.

● Hewson Brace (Seattle Seat)

A Hewson brace is made of foam and hard plastic with Velcro fasteners. It is used as a next step up from the Pavlik harness. Some doctors prescribe the Hewson brace after a spica cast is removed. This brace can usually be removed for bathing and changing diapers. Babies can learn to sit up while wearing this brace.

● Ilfeld Splint

An Ilfeld splint is used for younger children, sometimes when the Pavlik harness has not been effective (see Figure 29).

Tip: The cotton straps and pads on an Ilfeld splint are washable. Ask for an extra pair of each from your orthotist. When you want to wash the straps, put the clean extra pair onto the brace. Then put the worn straps into the washing machine. Use mild soap or detergent and dry the straps completely before you put them back on. If you change the pads, do so one at a time because the cuffs are not marked left and right.

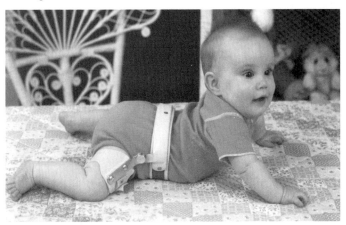

FIGURE 29. A baby wearing an Ilfeld splint *(Photo courtesy of Fillauer, LLC)*

Typically, you can remove the Ilfeld splint to bathe your child and for diaper changes. The brace goes on top of clothing. When dressing your child, make sure that no wrinkles are under the splint, as this can irritate the skin. Some parents apply moleskin to the back of the brace in the hard plastic areas. Moleskin is sold in drugstores in the section with foot care products. Use scissors to cut it to the right size, and then apply the adhesive backing to the brace.

◉ Hip Abduction Splints

You will find a number of different braces called hip abduction splints. The brace shown in Figure 30 comes in two models, one of which is adjustable.

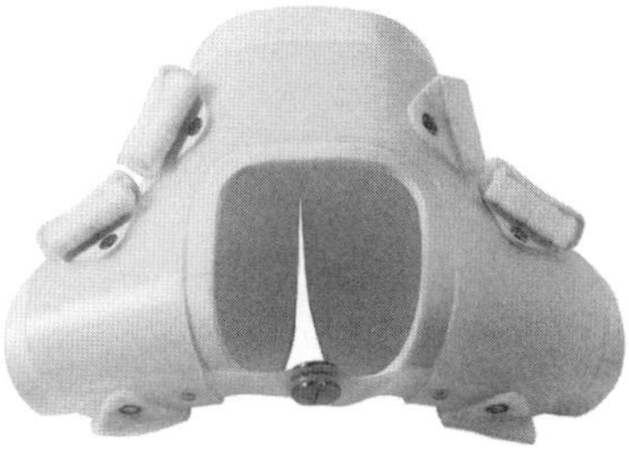

FIGURE 30. A hip abduction splint *(Photo courtesy of Trulife)*

Another type of brace is the dynamic hip splint (see Figure 31). It is worn over clothing and can be adjusted as a child grows.

Two splints that are uncommon in the United States are the Craig splint (also called the Aberdeen splint) and the Von Roson splint. The plastic Craig splint is worn on top of a diaper and has loop-and-hook (Velcro) fasteners. It is removed for diaper changes and can be wiped off with a cloth if it needs to be cleaned. The Von Roson splint should be removed only by a doctor. For more information about these splints, see *The STEPS Splint Book*, by Sue Banton and Tracy Brader, available at the Steps Charity website, www.steps-charity.org.uk.

● Rhino Cruiser Brace

The Rhino Cruiser brace can be used by babies and children up to three years old. It comes in five different sizes. A child can wear it while walking (see Figure 32).

Tip: For a Rhino Cruiser brace, if the foam on the brace is too long, it might slip out. Usually fasteners come with this brace. Check

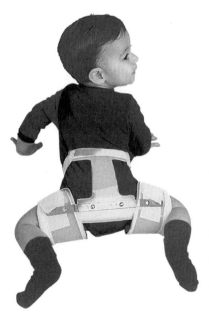

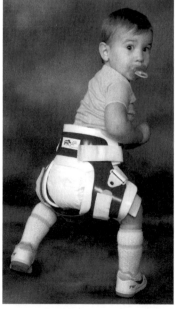

FIGURE 32. A child fitted in a Rhino Cruiser brace *(Photo courtesy of Rhino Pediatric Orthopedic Designs, Inc.)*

FIGURE 31. A child wearing a dynamic hip splint *(Photo courtesy of Trulife)*

the package contents. You can use the fasteners to adjust the extra foam. This should solve the problem.

● Scottish Rite Brace (Atlanta Brace)

This brace is often used with older children who are already walking or old enough to walk. It is called a walking abduction brace. It has hinges at the top that allow the child's legs to move back and forth but not from side to side. This brace is worn on top of clothing. You can remove the brace to bathe your child, and you can clean the cuffs of the brace by wiping them with a damp washcloth.

● Wheaton Brace

The Wheaton brace is made of foam and plastic. It comes in five sizes and resembles the brace shown in Figure 33. To see an actual photo of the brace and read its product description, see the website www .wheatonbrace.com/products/whao.html.

● Fitting a Brace

After the doctor prescribes a brace, your child is scheduled for two appointments at an orthotics facility. During the first visit, the orthotist measures your child to determine the right-size brace. Though the doctor specifies which brace to use, most come in different sizes. At the second visit, the orthotist fits the brace to your child, making any adjustments that are needed to customize the fit.

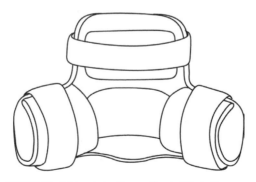

FIGURE 33. A hip abduction orthosis *(Illustration courtesy of Orthomerica Products, Inc.)*

The leg cuffs should be tight enough to keep the legs apart (abducted), but not so tight that they irritate the child's skin. The orthotist can show you how to check the skin pressure to make sure that your child stays comfortable. When the brace is properly fitted, it should stay in place when the baby moves his or her legs, even if the baby tries to squeeze them together. The orthotist shows you how to adjust the brace, how to remove it, and how to put it back on.

When a child is outgrowing a brace, the abdominal strap gets too tight. If the brace has foam materials, the foam leg wrap might slip out of place. The child could be fussy, especially if he or she has gas or needs to be burped. The baby might not sleep as well at night. Let the doctor know that you think he or she needs a bigger brace. If your child figures out how to remove the brace, you can use Velcro fasteners to hold the straps around the back and out of reach.

Car Seats—You Might Need a New One

You might not know whether you need a different car seat until after your child is fitted with a brace. If your child doesn't fit into your car seat, then remove the brace for the car ride home from the doctor's office. Put your child in the car seat without the brace so that he or she can ride home safely. Then take your child and the brace to a store with lots of car seats options. Put the brace on your child and try them out. Select a car seat with low sides. Some children fit well into convertible car seats with low sides. The specific brand does not matter. The most important consideration is how your child fits into the seat while wearing the brace.

If your doctor allows your child time during the day to go without a brace, then your child can ride in a car seat without it. But then you'll need to keep track of how long the child spends in the car seat so that the time does not exceed the amount that is allowed.

A Brace at Home

When a child first starts wearing a brace, he or she might be fussy while getting used to it. Typically, pain medication is not needed. If you are concerned that your child is in pain, contact your doctor.

It is very important for the child to wear the brace consistently for the number of hours that the doctor specified. Otherwise his or her hips might not get better. If your child is wearing a brace after having a cast removed, see "When the Cast Comes Off" on page 150 for more information about this adjustment period.

Usually the brace can be removed for diaper changes. The first few times it might take you a little while to figure out how the straps go back on. This gets easier with practice. If your baby wears a Hewson brace, make sure that the diaper does not have any creases or folds because the brace will press them into the skin. If your child wears the brace 24 hours a day, you might be allowed to remove it to give your child a bath for half an hour every other day or so. If your child's brace is washable, make sure to keep it clean by washing it periodically for your child's comfort.

◉ Diapering

Due to the position of your child's legs when wearing the brace, you might discover that her diaper leaks more than before during naps or at night. You can use an incontinence pad such as Depends or Poise inside the diaper to solve this problem.

Tip: For a boy, incontinence pads might not work because he needs more room in the front, and also the pads in front might get too full too fast. Try a diaper that is wide in the crotch area such as Pampers Swaddlers New Baby diapers. If you use Pampers diapers, make sure the cartoon character cannot be seen on the front side. For Huggies diapers, make sure the character is centered over his penis.

◉ Potty Training in a Brace

If your child is the right age for potty training and he or she is wearing a brace, you should still be able to go ahead with the potty training. The brace keeps the hips flexed up and the thighs spread apart, which is a position that also works well when sitting on the toilet. Keep a close watch on your child to make sure that he or she stays in this position. After your child has finished and is cleaned up, put the brace back on. If you have any worries or concerns, contact your child's doctor and explain the situation.

● Skin Care

To avoid skin irritation, wash your child's skin twice daily and wash any plastic foam twice daily as well. Check your child's skin when the brace is removed. If there is redness that lasts longer than one hour, the brace should be adjusted by the orthotist.

● Clothing Tips

Some children get rashes from the foam on the brace if it rubs against their skin. To keep this from happening, dress the child so that the legs are covered before you put on the brace. For daytime, you can use tights or leggings, or boys' tube socks with the toes cut out—pull them up the legs to go under the brace.

On top of the brace, a onesie with pants or sweat pants can work. For girls, you can try a one-piece romper outfit or dresses to cover the brace.

At nighttime, pajamas that snap on the inside of the legs work well. If you buy them two or three sizes too large, then you can snap them around the brace. Footed pajamas with wide openings (zippers down to the toes on one leg) also work. For some braces, thin cotton pajamas can be worn under the brace.

Securing the Straps on a Brace

Some babies tug on the brace straps or figure out how to take off a brace. Here are some suggestions about how to secure the straps:

* Safety pins. For a Rhino Cruiser brace, safety pins or diaper pins can work in a pinch, but could damage the straps over time.

* Medical tape. Tape down the straps. Some doctors put tape on the adjustment straps.

* Clothing. If the weather is cool, cover the straps with clothes. For some braces such as a Rhino Cruiser brace, you might be able to put lightweight pants on top of it.

* Metal rings on the straps. The orthotist can add a metal ring around the Velcro section of each strap. Then the child can open only the end portion of the straps.

If you discover your child gleefully running laps around the coffee table with the brace held over his head, talk to the doctor. The doctor might agree to limit the brace to nap time or bedtime depending on the condition of the child's hips. If that is not possible, discuss ways to secure the brace so that the child cannot remove it. One orthotist suggests that parents be "kindly persistent" explaining to the child that the brace is "good" for the child's legs and hips, which is why the doctor prescribed it.

How a Child Moves in a Brace

Children can sit in the brace and learn to sit, roll over, crawl, walk, and climb. When sleeping, children can easily move around and can lie on their stomachs or on the side with one leg in the air. Older children might remove the brace. Check to see if the brace needs to be put back on after your child has settled at nap time or at night. Some suggestions to encourage movement are included here.

Rolling. To encourage a young baby to roll, prop him or her up at the waist with a pillow. He or she might find it easier to learn how to roll from this position. Some children can roll from tummy to back, but not the reverse.

Crawling. If your child is crawling, protect his or her knees and the tops of the feet. The crawl will be different than usual due to the angle of the hips. Use pants that cover the knees, or use tube socks with the toes cut out. If the straps bother your child, make sure that he or she wears something under the straps so that they do not rub against the skin and cause irritation.

Standing and walking. If a child wants to stand, let him or her figure out how to pull up. If your child is not pulling up and is the right age for it, then you might want to try a baby walker to get the child used to the idea of using his or her legs and trying to stand. Older children can walk in the brace and even go up stairs.

Here is one mother's story of a major milestone. Her daughter, Jemma, learned to stand in a brace. Jemma had a closed reduction and wore a cast, which was then followed by a brace:

Our wee girl Jemma is now nearly fourteen months, and yesterday she stood for the first time. I was trying to have a sleep at the time (ten weeks until Baby Number Two arrives), and my husband came pounding up the stairs shouting, "Are you awake?"

Well, I was then! He was so excited (and great Dad got to see something first). He dragged me down the stairs to see, and sure enough, she was pulling herself up onto her feet and holding on for dear life. She's since done it a few more times, so I guess walking will be her next big achievement (and a new round of baby-proofing the house!).   [TRINA]

Checkups for a Child Wearing a Brace

The doctor tells you how often the baby or child needs to be checked while wearing the brace. During the checkup, the doctor examines your child's hips. An ultrasound or X rays are taken at some visits so that the doctor can see how your child's hip joints are developing.

If your child's hips are not improving while wearing a brace, the doctor either continues to monitor the hips or changes the treatment plan. Some treatments work best when a child is at a specific age. If this is the case, the doctor should be able to explain this to you. If you are concerned about your child's treatment, consider getting a second opinion from a different pediatric orthopedic doctor.

An older child (four to six years old) might wear the Scottish Rite brace. Sometimes the child can choose the color of the straps and the design of the cuffs. One child who was diagnosed at age four wore a cast for five months and then was fitted with a Scottish Rite brace. It took five days before she tried to walk in the brace. She wore the brace for eighteen months. During that time, she rode her bike and scooter, and ran and played. Her doctor placed a few limits on her activities—such as not jumping on a trampoline. The hardest part for this child was not the wearing of the brace; it was the fact that some people stared at her while she was wearing it. For suggestions about this topic, see "How Other People React to Your Child" on page 147.

When Treatment with the Brace Ends

Wearing the brace usually improves the child's hips. As the child's hips get better, he or she wears it for shorter lengths of time until it is no longer needed. Trina's daughter, Jemma, wore a brace after a cast. Her hips got better until only follow-up visits were needed, as explained in this quote.

> Jemma is now brace free. We had an X ray today and met with her specialist, who said her hips look "great." They are still totally stable, and the coverage of socket over the hip bone is a huge improvement from three months ago.... SO, he said she could be brace free and [that he would] see us again in six months.   **[TRINA]**

Many children are done with treatment after the brace and need only follow-up checkups. Others need surgery. For more information about the types of surgery used to treat hip dysplasia, see Chapter 7, "Surgical Treatments," beginning on page 100.

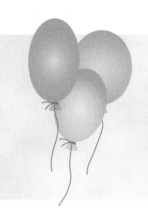

6

If Your Child Needs Surgery

For children who experienced hip dysplasia at a later age or did not respond to early treatment with a Pavlik harness or brace, surgery is used to correct hip dysplasia. Because children heal quickly and their bones are still developing, surgery can significantly improve the hip-joint structure. After surgery, children up to about six years of age typically wear casts. Older children and adolescents do not wear casts during recovery. This chapter describes how to prepare for surgery and what is involved in a typical surgery day and postoperative recovery.

Questions to Ask the Doctor

Asking the following questions might help you to better understand your child's surgery:

* What kind of surgery does my child need?
* What would be the best-case and the worst-case outcomes for this surgery?
* How long is the standard surgery?
* How many times have you performed this operation?
* Can I direct-donate blood for my child's operation if you anticipate the need?

* What kind of pain relief medicine will be given to my child during surgery and afterward?

* Can my child take a favorite toy to the operating room for comfort?

* When my child wakes up, how should I expect him or her to act?

* How long do you expect my child to stay in the hospital after surgery?

And if your child will wear a cast after the surgery, asking the following questions can help you prepare for it:

* How long will my child be in a cast after surgery?

* How many cast changes will there be?

* What shape and how wide will the cast be? (The doctor might not know the shape of the cast before the surgery, but if he does know, ask him to show you a picture or a drawing of it.)

* Are there any restrictions for my child afterward? Is it all right for my child to stand in the cast?

* If problems arise with my child's cast, whom do I call—the hospital or your office? Can I relate my question to the office staff, and will you call me back?

Talking with Your Child or Teen

It is best to tell children age two years or older that they are going to have surgery. For young children, use simple language that they can understand. One mother told her daughter that she had "a hip boo boo" that needed to be fixed. Explain that the surgery is what you want to do and that you will be nearby in the hospital.

A young child might like to make a cast for a doll or stuffed animal at home before he or she goes to the hospital. Some hospitals have programs where the child can visit to get used to the setting before the day of surgery. Children are shown the hospital gown, gas mask, and other equipment. If your child is much older (six years and up), take some time to explain the surgery to her or ask the doctor to explain it to her while you are present.

Vivian's daughter, Angela, was diagnosed with hip dysplasia at the age of five. She needed two surgeries to treat her bilateral hip dysplasia. Each surgery corrected one of Angela's hips. (For a link to a video about Angela, see "Online Video Resources" on page 189.) In the following quote, Vivian describes some of the emotional issues that came up with Angela before her second surgery:

> I think one of the more difficult things with an older child is that they are more aware of what's going on. This was especially true for this second surgery. She knew what was coming and was more anxious. She had nightmares and said she was scared. We explained that [the surgery] was so that she could have a pain-free future. We bought her worry dolls so that she could whisper her worries to them and they would "take them away" as she slept. I spoke with a counselor about how to handle this. I feel that it would be helpful to other parents to be aware of this aspect of hip dysplasia and older kids. **[VIVIAN]**

Preteens and teens can understand more than a young child. Adolescents can be more involved when the doctor explains treatment. Give your teen opportunities to talk about any worries or fears that he or she has and to ask questions. Explain ahead of time how many days the doctor expects the teen to stay at the hospital after the surgery, and about how many weeks or months that crutches or a walker will likely be needed. Even if the doctor has gone over this while your teen is present, it can be hard to absorb everything that is said. Discuss your plans for managing school assignments and returning to school. Also explain any restrictions that the hospital has about visits from friends or the use of cell phones.

Planning Ahead

Usually a child's surgery is scheduled weeks or months ahead of time. In the meantime, you can do some planning in advance that will make it easier to manage when your child is recovering from the surgery.

● *Planning the Trip Home and Riding in the Car*

If your child is young enough, you will need a car seat that your child can fit into while wearing the cast (see Figure 34). This can be hard to plan for, because the doctor might not know exactly what position the child's legs will be in until surgery. Each cast must fit the child individually, with the ideal position for each hip. One child's cast can have the legs positioned much wider apart than another.

Important: Never modify a car seat because that can affect the ability of the seat to protect your child in case of an accident. If you borrow or buy a used car seat, make sure that it has not already been in an accident. A car seat that has been in an accident is unsafe to use again.

If your child is wearing a cast, finding a car seat the right size and shape to fit your child can be a challenge. You might need to try out a number of car seats to find the best fit. Some convertible car seats with low sides and wide seats such as Britax models work. Ask your doctor or hospital about a car seat if your child is having surgery. Many hospitals can provide loaner or rental car seats, as they are often much more expensive than regular car seats and can cost $300 to $500. Some health-insurance plans cover this cost.

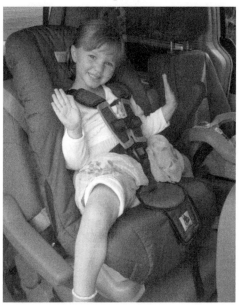

FIGURE 34.
Samantha riding in the car in a Snug Seat Hippo car seat
(Photo courtesy of Jason Skrinak)

A previous model from Snug Seat was the Spelcast convertible car seat. It is no longer in production but was also made to work with a spica cast. Some hospitals and fire departments might still have them available as loaners.

Children who are too big for a car seat but too young or too small to sit in the front seat can use an E-Z-ON vest to ride safely in the back seat while lying down. The E-Z-ON vest comes in a regular upright style and in a modified style. Two types are available—one zips up the back, and the other has push buttons on the front (see Figure 35). The zip-up type is a good choice for children who like to unbuckle themselves. To make your child comfortable, use pillows as needed under the head and under the legs.

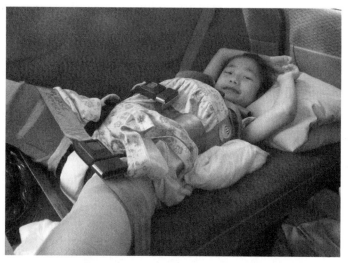

FIGURE 35. Megan, age seven, riding in the car wearing an E-Z-ON vest *(Photo courtesy of Patti Streeter)*

Adolescents who are old enough and large enough to sit in the front seat will not have a cast after surgery. Recline the front passenger seat so that your child is comfortable and the seatbelt can be fastened.

If your child has medical challenges beyond hip dysplasia, you might need to use a safety vest such as the E-Z-ON Safety Vest, or a car bed instead of a car seat. A car bed lets an infant travel lying down. These are needed when, for medical reasons, the child cannot sit. For more information about car seats, car beds, and the manufacturers who make them, contact the Automotive Safety Program. Contact information is listed in "Health and Medical Organizations" on page 190.

● *Temporary Disabled Person Parking Placards*

Consider arranging for a placard that will allow you to park in handicap parking places when your child is recovering from surgery. The placard is useful whether you have a baby or young child who will wear a cast or an older child who will be using a wheelchair and crutches or a walker. These parking spaces are located close to building entrances, and they have extra room on the sides so that you won't get pinned in by other cars parking too close for you to get your child out of the car.

> I applied for a temporary handicap placard from the DMV. I did this for both surgeries, and this is very helpful because having Angela in the wheelchair and a large family, getting a closer parking spot makes things much easier. I would suggest applying for it a few weeks before surgery since it takes several weeks to process—at least here in Massachusetts.   **[VIVIAN]**

The placard is good for up to six months. To get a temporary disabled parking placard, contact your state's department of motor vehicles (DMV). You will need to get a form for your child's doctor to sign. When you turn in the signed form at the DMV, you can get the placard. Follow the instructions from the DMV about where to put the placard in your car and when to use it. In some states, this is free. Other states charge a fee for the placard.

● *Making Arrangements at School*

Discuss with your doctor how long you should realistically plan for your child to miss school after surgery. If you are able to schedule surgery in the summer, your child might be able to return to school at the beginning of the school year either wearing a cast or using crutches or a walker (depending on the child's age). If the surgery is during the school year, you will need to allow enough rest and recovery time for your child.

Most public schools will send teachers to the home if children are expected to miss more than three weeks of school. The school might also be able to develop a plan in which the child attends school part-time. It is best to start the paperwork before surgery. Dr. Katherine Fan, a child and adolescent psychiatrist and pediatrician has this to say about working with schools:

> Some children and teens may benefit from a home school program. With the doctor's note, the family can request the school district to provide a more individualized and supportive learning plan in the comfort of home. This is especially helpful if the return to school coincides with the end of the school year, which tends to be more hectic and stressful.   [KATHERINE FAN, MD]

When your child does return to school either part-time or full-time, expect a lot of questions about what is wrong, especially if your child is wearing a cast or using crutches. Some schools are better able to accommodate students' needs than others. It is unlikely that your child's school has experience with hip dysplasia treatment. It can be helpful for the doctor to write a letter explaining what your child's needs are likely to be.

Megan was seven when she had surgery for hip dysplasia. Initially, her school suggested tutoring at home during the time she would be in a spica cast because the staff was concerned they would not be able to accommodate her needs. Megan's parents thought she would be better off at school. In response, the school asked for a letter from the doctor explaining what her needs would be after surgery. After the school received the letter, Megan was allowed to attend school while she was still wearing a spica cast. She used a pediatric reclining wheelchair. Megan's mother, Patti, describes their school situation in the following quote:

Megan did attend school while in the spica cast. We have the advantage that she attends a small Christian school, where I also teach. We were required to provide a letter from [Megan's doctor] stating what care would be required for her to be in school. She spent the day in the reclining wheelchair. We only reclined it part way. Her desk was turned sideways next to the wheelchair. She used a clipboard for writing assignments. Reading was no problem. She kept a sipper cup of water on her desk each day, since it was difficult to use the water fountain.

At lunch time we pulled her wheelchair to the end of the lunch table and put the back of the chair fully upright. I would reposition her so that she could be more upright to eat. When lunch was over, I reclined the chair again. She often went outside for recess, so that she could at least be outside and with the other children. Sometimes she read or played with toys; sometimes she would toss a ball with one of her friends. Her classmates handled the whole experience beautifully and were very helpful and understanding.   **[PATTI]**

While most people do not work at the same school their children attend, many schools do have aides or other staff who can assist children who have medical needs.

Lisa had several childhood surgeries for hip dysplasia. When she was twelve, Lisa had a PAO surgery on her left hip. This is what she remembers about starting seventh grade on crutches.

I had the surgery in June, so I started seventh grade at a new school that was under construction while on crutches and having no locker. Getting around school was a little challenging. There were only stairs: no elevators were available. Most other students were curious: asking what happened, staring, etc. It seems like a lot of people automatically assume you are on crutches due to an accident instead of a congenital condition.

Academically I did well. Socially, it was more challenging. I wanted to do what all my friends were doing—go to football games, a Halloween party, and on a hayride. My mom was so afraid I would get hurt that she didn't want to let me be "normal." That was the challenging part. As a kid, you want to fit in. I spent my whole teen years trying to prove to my family as well as myself that I was normal. I played softball (as a catcher believe it or not) to prove I could do it. In some ways, although it was difficult, it made me who I am today. I am goal oriented, and you better believe that if someone says I can't do something, I will prove them wrong. I owe that determination to my dysplasia. It pushed me to succeed.   **[LISA]**

Happy Hips, a group of teens with hip dysplasia, has the following to say about how surgery can affect school for teens:

Teenagers face many challenges including examinations, relationships, and personal or external pressures. These increase when you place surgery into the equation. Surgery takes a lot of energy out of anyone and has an unwanted effect on concentration. Firstly, there is the pain in the hip area, which is controlled by strong painkillers that can cause side effects including drowsiness that decrease your attention span. This makes school extremely hard as, sadly, the teachers cannot change certain deadlines or examination dates [such as A levels or AP exams]. It is extremely important for the teenager, his or her family, and the school to have strong links and to be in constant contact as needed.

It is clear from our members that teenagers struggle to tell their friends and classmates about upcoming surgery or about their condition. In the majority of cases, they have expressed their worries to teachers who have then been able to tell their classmates as a group and inform them how important their support is.

Secondly, there is the stress of not being able to concentrate all of the time. The most important thing is that parents are supportive of their children. Sometimes teens need a quick after-school nap for an hour before facing their homework.

On the other hand, it is extremely important to keep up with schoolwork, and it is evident that some parents feel that they are being hard on their children when they have to keep checking up on them. Our founder has personally been through this experience herself during her A levels [formal exams]. **[THE HAPPY HIPS TEAM]**

● *Taking Time Off from Work*

In the United States, depending on the size of the company where you work, the Family Medical Leave Act (FMLA) might allow you to take up to 12 weeks unpaid leave per year to care for a family member. As mentioned, this is the same act that covers maternity leave. This can be helpful if a child needs surgery. If your child is already attending day care, he or she can continue during treatment after recovering from surgery. See "Child Care" on page 49.

Preoperative Appointment

A preoperative (pre-op) appointment is scheduled for two or three weeks before your child's surgery. At this appointment, your child is checked to make sure that he or she is healthy enough for surgery.

During this visit, the doctor examines the child and goes over the planned surgery with you and your child if he or she is old enough to understand the conversation. Your child might have some tests. You might be told to stop any medications that your child is taking, and you might be given instructions about what he or she should eat in the days before the surgery. Some pediatric departments are set up to show children around before surgery or to provide coloring books to help them understand what to expect. Hospitals provide parents with a pre-op packet of information that has instructions for when to bring the child in for surgery, where to park, and which forms need to be filled out.

You will be given instructions about how to prepare your child for surgery. For example, your child might not be able to eat prior to the surgery. Many doctors consider breast milk to be a clear liquid, which is allowed up to four hours before surgery even if the child cannot eat food. Find out if your child can be scheduled for surgery early in the day: this can make it easier to manage withholding food.

If your child will wear a cast, ask your child's doctor about the cast materials (fiberglass or plaster) so that you know what to expect.

Ask if it is possible for you to speak with another parent whose child has undergone similar surgery for hip dysplasia.

Ask about how to safely drive your child home after surgery, and if the hospital has a car seat loaner program if your child is young enough to need a car seat.

For more information about casts, see Chapter 8, "Caring for a Child in a Cast," beginning on page 121.

Surgery Day

This section gives an overview of what typically happens on the day that a child has orthopedic surgery. The Hospital for Special Surgery (HSS) has an excellent video that describes this process (www.hss.edu/pediatric-orthopedic-surgery.asp). The video is specifically about HSS, so some details might be different from your experience, but it may still be informative. Before the surgery day, you should follow the instructions that the hospital provided to withhold food and or liquids from your child.

Generally, this is what happens:

* Your child is checked into the hospital for surgery. This process varies depending on the hospital, but typically the hospital staff asks about your child's health history, allergies, and past reaction to medications. Your child is given a hospital gown to wear and an ID bracelet.

* The doctor examines your child to make sure that she is still healthy enough for surgery.

* Next, the doctor goes over the surgery with you. Your child will be included in this conversation if she is old enough to understand what is going on.

* Anesthesia is given to your child to put her to sleep.

* You are told where you can wait during the surgery. Your child remains asleep in the operating room (OR) throughout the surgery.

* Your child is moved to a recovery area to wake up. You might be able to sit with her.

* If your child will need to stay overnight, the hospital staff moves your child into a room. Usually, a parent can stay overnight with the child.

* How long your child stays at the hospital depends on what kind of surgery is performed and how she responds to the surgery.

◉ *What to Bring to the Hospital*

For the day of surgery and, possibly, an overnight stay, you may need a number of items. Regardless of the length of stay, always keep the most important items with you. If your child will be staying overnight, pack a bag and leave it in the car until after the surgery. When your child has a room, get the bag out of the car, or ask someone to bring it to you. The following sections offer suggestions about what to bring when you go to the hospital.

For Babies and Young Children
These items should fit into most diaper bags:

* Your child's favorite blanket or stuffed animal.

* Extra pacifiers if your child uses them.

* Snacks such as crackers and juice boxes or a sippy cup for your child.

* Diapering supplies, regular size to use before surgery.

* Diapering supplies to use with the cast: small (size 1) diapers to go inside the cast, plus large (size 5) diapers to go outside the cast. Some parents also use incontinence pads (Depends or Poise) inside the cast.

If your child is in traction at the hospital, or needs surgery that will require him or her to stay overnight, bring these items:

* Child's clothing. Bring socks, a shirt, pajama top, or nightgown one size larger to go over a cast, and shoes if your child wears them.

* New books or toys for child. Your child might enjoy a balloon from the hospital gift shop. If you have a portable DVD player, bring it along with some favorite movies.

* If you are also staying overnight, bring comfortable clothes for yourself. Sweats work well for nighttime. Also bring a towel, slippers, snacks, and a book, magazine, or laptop computer. If you are breast-feeding, consider bringing a pump.

* Some parents bring a box of candy for the nurses and staff members. If you want to take pictures, bring your camera.

Note: If you bring valuables with you to the hospital keep an eye on them as thefts can occur.

For Preteens and Teens

Older children and teens often like to bring an iPod or MP3 player so that they can listen to music. Handheld game consoles are also popular. If your child wants to bring a cell phone, check with the hospital to find out what the policy is for cell phones. Books and magazines are also good, though it might take some time after surgery before your child feels well enough to enjoy reading. Also follow the hospital's recommendations about valuables.

Preteens and teenagers typically stay in the children's ward, along with younger children. Even if a teen is adult-size, pediatric facilities are best equipped to manage their surgery. When it comes to osteotomies, even adults sometimes are seen by pediatric orthopedic surgeons because they are more likely to have specialized knowledge about this surgery.

In Your Purse or Wallet

These items are helpful in getting through the hospital paperwork and passing the time while your child is in surgery.

* Your photo ID.
* A folder with insurance cards, referrals, and medical information.
* A cellular (mobile) phone or change for a pay phone, and a list of phone numbers of friends and family to call after the surgery.
* Snacks or change for vending machines.
* A book, magazine, or deck of cards.

● Anesthesia

Before surgery, the child is given anesthesia for pain relief and to put him or her to sleep. Your child could be given either gas or an IV. He or she might also have an epidural. A pediatric anesthesiologist usually handles pain relief when a child has surgery. These doctors have special training to work with babies and children. Some hospitals allow a parent to take the child to the operating room.

Though the idea of anesthesia for your child can be scary, keep in mind that most children who have surgery for hip dysplasia (or other orthopedic surgery), are otherwise healthy. This means that they are in the group of patients who are considered the most fit for surgery. The American Society of Anesthesiologists (ASA) uses a physical classification system for assessing fitness for surgery from 1 to 6, with 1 being the most fit. If your child has additional medical concerns besides hip dysplasia, the anesthesiologist takes these into consideration.

If an older child is very scared about the surgery, he or she could be given a "cocktail" such as liquid diazepam (Valium) to calm him or her down first. For a longer procedure, children two years of age or older might also be given some medicine to prevent nausea and vomiting during recovery. Usually these medicines are not needed for younger babies. Young babies are less likely to be scared or to have nausea or vomiting after surgery. If your child is under two and has had nausea or vomiting after anesthesia in the past, tell the doctor, and ask for medicine to help keep it from happening again.

Note: Sometimes the cocktail and antinausea medicines are not given before very short procedures, such as cast changes. This is because the effects can last longer than the procedure. If the child is still groggy from the cocktail, it can complicate his or her recovery.

Epidural

For some surgeries, an epidural is used in addition to general anesthesia. An epidural is pain medicine that numbs and blocks pain; it is given through a soft tube called a catheter into the epidural space, which is near the backbone and spinal cord. The pediatric anesthesiologist uses a needle to insert the epidural and then tapes the tube so that it stays in place during surgery. The medicine comes from an epidural pump on a pole near the bed. With the epidural, a smaller dose of pain relief medicine can be used for just the right area of your child's body. A smaller dose of medicine can reduce side effects because less general anesthesia is needed. Sometimes the anesthesiologist places the epidural before surgery while the child is in the operating room (OR).

Note: With an epidural, there is the chance that it will not provide complete pain relief (some women have this problem during childbirth). The pediatric anesthesiologist can adjust the pain relief medicine if this happens.

An epidural provides pain relief for several hours after surgery and can let the muscles relax, which reduces muscle spasms. For a surgery in which the child will remain in the hospital overnight, the epidural might be left in place until the child can tolerate oral pain medicine. When your child can eat and drink, typically he or she is given medicine orally (by mouth), and the IV or epidural medication is stopped. Often the pediatric anesthesiologist continues to be involved after the surgery to help with pain management. Ask if this is the case at your hospital.

Your child might be sore for the first few days and could have muscle spasms. More pain medicine and muscle relaxants might be ordered. Typically, your child's doctor writes which medicines are allowed on your child's medical chart. This is so that you will not have to find the doctor if your child is in pain.

Spinal Block

A spinal block is an injection into the spine that provides pain relief from the waist down. It is similar to an epidural, except that the epidural can be left in place so that pain medicine can be administered over a longer period of time.

● Coping with Your Child's Surgical Treatment

The following quote eloquently expresses one mother's feelings about her daughter's surgery for hip dysplasia:

> Lots of people say, "It's not a big deal," or "She won't remember it." But mothers remember everything. I was haunted by the memory of my daughter being carried away by the nurses when she went in for surgery. I felt like a terrible mother because my daughter smiled and went willingly, trusting that I would not put her in harm's way. It broke my heart to know that she would wake up in the spica.
>
> ➡

It was hard to keep in the front of my heart that I was doing this to care for and protect my daughter. To know in your head and know in your heart are two different things.

Mine went in at nine months old, and she is three [years old] now. When I see her running around the playground with no limp or hindrance, I am glad for what happened. When she goes in for checkups, and I see fourteen-year-old girls who walk with difficulty down the hall to see the orthopedic specialist, I am thankful for the spica. But it has taken time for me to be grateful in my heart and not just in the logical part of my head. [HIP-BABY DISCUSSION GROUP]

Even though you know it is coming, the sight of your child going into surgery and the first time you see your child afterward can be very hard. Do what you can to mentally prepare yourself and get as much support as you can from family and friends.

Postoperative (Post-Op) Recovery at the Hospital

The length of time that your child stays at the hospital depends on the type of surgery involved and the rate at which the individual child heals. The doctor and hospital staff will manage pain relief and inflammation and check your child's progress to make sure that he or she is ready to go home before being discharged from the hospital.

Babies and Young Children

Your child might be able to come home from the hospital within hours after a closed reduction, or he may need to stay for a day or two after an open reduction or osteotomy. During this time, pain medicine is needed. Your child's doctor writes instructions on your child's chart for pain relief. This can avoid delays if medicine is needed when the anesthesia wears off. If your doctor gives you a prescription, fill it at the hospital pharmacy if possible. You can avoid a possible delay in case your local pharmacy doesn't have the medicine.

For a surgery in which the child remains in the hospital over-night, an epidural might be left in place until the child can tolerate oral pain medicine. When your child can eat and drink, typically he is given medicine orally (by mouth), and the IV or epidural medication is stopped. For information about pain management after your child leaves the hospital, see "Pain Management at Home" on page 97.

Take whatever supplies the nurses give you, such as moleskin and waterproof tape for a cast. Even if you can't use them right away, they will come in handy later when you are at home. It's a good idea to change your child's diaper before you leave the hospital. This gives you a chance to manage a diaper change with a spica cast where sup-port is available if you need it. This also can prevent the child's diaper from leaking into the cast on the way home.

Tip: After surgery, your child might be given a device called an incentive spirometer to help clear out his chest from the anesthesia. This expands the lungs to prevent pneumonia. If your child hesitates, does not know what to do, or is afraid, ask about using a familiar toy such as a pinwheel or bubbles instead. For example, if a child can blow 10 bubbles an hour, that works as well as the incentive spiro-meter.

● *Older Children and Adolescents*

Older children and teens do not wear a cast after surgery, and they might need to stay in the hospital for up to a week. A hospital stay af-ter a PAO is usually five to seven days. Typically, an epidural is left in place after surgery, and your child will also have an IV and a catheter. Your child will probably receive pain medication through a pump. The child presses a button to get more medicine as needed. This is called a patient-controlled anesthesia (PCA). When your child can eat and drink, he or she is given medicine orally (by mouth), and the IV or epidural medication is stopped. Cold therapy might be used in which a nurse or other health-care worker puts ice on your child's hip to ease pain and inflammation.

Older children and teens need physical therapy after an oste-otomy. Very soon after surgery, a physical therapist begins teaching your child exercises and, as tolerated, how to get in and out of bed and how to use crutches or a walker. Your child might also be taught how to use a wheelchair.

It could be months after the surgery before an adolescent can bear full weight on the hip that had the osteotomy. This might seem overwhelming, but one thing to keep in mind is that teens heal faster after hip surgery than adults do. In other words, if your child waits until adulthood to have this surgery, it will take longer for him or her to recover.

Your teen might use a continuous passive motion (CPM) machine during recovery. A CPM machine moves the hip joint without any effort from the child. This can be less painful for the child than trying to move the hip joint on his or her own. Moving the hip joint during recovery is important to keep the hip from becoming stiff and to limit the amount of scar tissue that forms.

Side Effects and Complications

A side effect is a secondary effect that can be caused by medical treatment. For instance, many of the strong pain relief medicines that are needed for surgery are known to have the side effect of constipation. A complication is an extra medical problem that is connected to a medical problem that already exists. A complication can be caused by the first medical problem or it can occur during treatment. For example, arthritis is a complication associated with untreated hip dysplasia; and infection could be a complication of surgery.

Doctors and the hospital staff make an effort to minimize the risk of side effects and complications, and to treat any problems that arise after surgery. Some common side effects during recovery are the inability to pee (urinary retention) and constipation. Potential complications specific to hip surgery are a leg-length discrepancy or numbness. Complications for surgery in general are allergic reactions, infection, pain, and blood clots.

Teens might wear compression stockings, often called TEDS (because of the brand name), after surgery to reduce the risk of blood clots. A blood clot that forms in a deep vein is called a deep vein thrombosis (DVT). A DVT can be painful and can create a health risk if it breaks off and travels through the bloodstream to the lungs. Babies and young children do not need to wear compression stockings.

● Swelling

Swelling is common after surgery. If your child has a cast, it might be tight for a few days until the swelling goes down. This can make diapering difficult at first. If your child is uncomfortable, the doctor might be able to make some cuts in the cast to relieve the pressure. Some casts include a window located over the child's stomach. This gives the stomach room to expand when the child eats. For older children who have had a pelvic osteotomy and are not casted, ice packs can help reduce swelling and alleviate pain.

● Muscle Spasms

During the first few days after surgery, your child might have muscle spasms. One mother described her daughter's muscle spasms this way:

> A few hours after surgery, she would scream in pain, start to drop off to sleep, and then scream again. It was terrifying. The nurse said that she was having muscle spasms, so they gave her [pain medication], and it worked.   **[HIP-BABY DISCUSSION GROUP]**

If a child has muscle spasms, pain medicine such as acetaminophen with codeine (Tylenol with codeine) or diazepam (Valium) is given to treat the spasms. Pain medicine might also be needed, but if the spasms are controlled, this decreases pain. Moving the child's feet during the day can help minimize spasms. Some parents have seen improvement at home if a child uses a beanbag chair during the day because it supports the child's weight evenly.

Leaving the Hospital

Your child's doctor decides when your child is ready to go home. Some considerations are that the child is healing, his or her pain is well managed, and, for an older child, he or she knows how to use the walking aid that the doctor prescribed.

You might want to check the following things before you leave:

* Have you filled your child's prescription for pain-relief medicine? Do you know when to give your child the next dose?

* Do you understand how your child should safely ride in the car? If you are unsure, ask about the car seat, restraint, or seat belts that will work for your child. If you have an older child or teen who is not wearing a cast, the staff can show you how to help your child into the car.

* Are you aware of any special symptoms that you should watch for at home? You might be given instructions about what symptoms to expect and in which situations you should call the doctor.

* If your child wears diapers, have you tried a diaper change with the cast? If not, change your child's diaper before you go home. That way, if you have questions, you can ask for advice.

* If your child has a cast, are the edges petalled with water-resistant tape?

* Have you gathered up all of your belongings and your child's belongings?

* Do you have all paperwork that the doctor provided to you such as prescriptions, a form for a temporary disabled parking placard, and a doctor's note for school?

* Have you scheduled your child's next doctor visit?

Pain Management at Home

After surgery, your doctor develops a pain management plan for your child. If your child is in pain, try to stay calm. This reduces his or her anxiety, and helps you focus on determining the source and intensity of the pain. Contact your doctor if you believe that your child's pain relief medicine needs to be adjusted.

If your child is old enough, ask if he or she is in pain, where it hurts, and how much it hurts. For babies or very young children, use behavior and appearance as a guide. A child's age and personality affect how he or she reacts to pain. One child might be very quiet, while another screams. Children in pain usually want to stay closer than usual to a parent or primary caregiver. Try to make yourself available. For example, put the baby where he or she can see you while you make dinner.

Pain can be treated with nonmedical techniques, such as distraction. Distraction can be as simple as allowing a child to watch more television than usual, playing music that he or she likes, reading a story together. For a baby, try breast-feeding (see "Breast-Feeding" on page 133).

The most common over-the-counter pain relief medications for children are acetaminophen (Tylenol) and ibuprofen (Advil or Motrin). Do not combine these medications unless your doctor has given you instructions to do so.

Acetaminophen provides pain relief for mild to moderate pain and fever. It does not relieve inflammation. Overdosing a child with acetaminophen can damage the liver and kidneys. Acetaminophen is included in many cough or cold medicines. Read medicine labels carefully to avoid accidentally giving your child too much acetaminophen. Make sure that you have the right-size teaspoon or dropper.

Ibuprofen is a nonsteroidal anti-inflammatory drug (NSAID). It reduces inflammation, provides pain relief, and reduces fevers. Ibuprofen prevents the body from making prostaglandins (hormones that produce inflammation and pain). As a side effect, ibuprofen can cause stomach irritation. It is best to take ibuprofen on a full stomach. If your child is allergic to aspirin or has asthma, check with your doctor before giving your child ibuprofen.

Aspirin is not recommended for babies or children unless directed by a doctor. Aspirin use in children is linked to a rare but serious disease called Reye's syndrome. Naproxen (Aleve, Naprosyn, or Anaprox) is recommended only for children who are at least twelve years old.

Some prescription pain relievers for children are acetaminophen with codeine (Tylenol with codeine) and hydrocodone with acetaminophen (Vicodin, Anexsia, Lorcet, or Norco). These medications can work very well to relieve pain, but since they are opiates, they also can make the child sleepy and constipated. Make sure that you keep them out of reach of children and throw away the medication after your child is better. They can be dangerous if overused. Your pharmacist can give you instructions for safe disposal of medication. Guidelines are also available on the website for the Institute for Safe Medication Practices at www.ismp.org (search for "throw away medicine").

If your child is taking acetaminophen with codeine and is not getting enough pain relief, notify your doctor. About 10 percent of people do not metabolize codeine effectively because their bodies do not break it down into the substances that relieve pain. If this is the case for your child, the doctor can prescribe a different medicine.

If stronger pain relief is needed, such as after an osteotomy, the doctor might prescribe a medicine such as oxycodone (Oxydose) for the child. If the child is very anxious, then lorazepam (Ativan) might be prescribed at bedtime to help him or her sleep.

How much pain medicine a baby or child needs depends on the child's weight. Make sure that you have a medication made for the size of your child. If you have a baby, use infant medication. This is safer for the baby and protects against overdosing. Read the label carefully. If you do not understand it, ask a pharmacist. They are trained to explain medication and can help you understand the proper dosage for your child. Once you know the right dose, you must measure it accurately. A household teaspoon might not be accurate. Check with your pharmacist about the best device for measuring liquid medicines.

After surgery, your child's pain should decrease each day. If there is a sudden increase in pain and you do not know why, contact your doctor's office for advice.

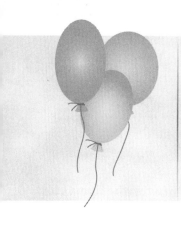

7

Surgical Treatments

As discussed in the previous chapter, for some children with hip dysplasia a nonsurgical treatment is not the answer. Perhaps the Pavlik harness or brace is unable to correct their hip dysplasia. Maybe they were too old for these nonsurgical treatments when the condition was diagnosed. When this is the case, a pediatric orthopedic surgeon performs surgery to correct the hip dysplasia, and there are several procedures he or she will consider. For all the surgical treatments described in this chapter, the child is put to sleep with anesthesia.

When possible, surgery to correct hip dysplasia is done during childhood. Because children heal quickly, and the bones are still developing, surgery can significantly improve the hip-joint structure. Even if an older teen has finished growing, as a young person his or her recovery will typically progress faster than that of an adult. After surgery, a child up to about six years old wears a cast, though some doctors use casts for children up to the age of ten.

Reduction

The most common type of surgery to treat babies and toddlers with hip dysplasia is a reduction, in which the doctor moves the ball at the top of the thighbone (femoral head) into the correct position inside the hip socket (acetabulum). Some children have traction before a reduction. Traction is a system of weights and pulleys used to gently stretch the muscles and tendons around the hip joint. See "Traction Before Surgery" on page 103.

Immediately before the reduction, the child is put to sleep with anesthesia and an arthrogram (X ray with dye) is taken. The doctor performs the surgery and applies a spica cast. This is a body cast that covers the child's torso and part or all of the legs. Another arthrogram is taken to confirm the position of the hip joint.

A child might have a closed reduction or an open reduction.

● Closed Reduction Surgery

The doctor is able to get the joint into the correct position without surgically opening the hip joint.

● Open Reduction Surgery

The doctor must surgically open the joint in order to get the femoral head in the correct position inside the hip socket.

The doctor might not know whether the surgery will be a closed or an open reduction until the surgery day when he or she sees the arthrogram images. Different types of open reductions have medical names based on the technique that the doctor uses. For example, a doctor can use a medial approach or anterolateral approach.

Medial Approach

If the child has bilateral hip dysplasia, both hips can be reduced at the same time. A study about this method, the "Systematic Review of Medial Open Reduction of the Hip," is currently underway (for information about the study, contact the International Hip Dysplasia Institute [IHDI]). The study will evaluate the long-term effectiveness of this surgery and the risk of avascular necrosis (AVN) as a complication. AVN is explained later in this chapter.

Anterolateral Approach (Also Called Smith-Peterson Approach)

This is often used with older children. Some facilities are experimenting with the use of ultrasound after the child is in a cast instead of an arthrogram (X ray with dye). The ultrasound is used to check

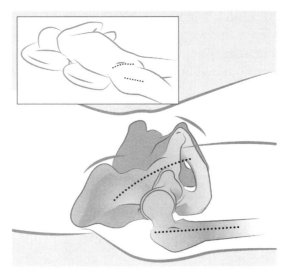

FIGURE 36. A Smith-Peterson open reduction (an anterolateral approach)

the hip position and the blood flow to the hip in the operating room after the cast is on the child (see Figure 36). It is difficult to get the ultrasound probe inside the cast for an accurate reading, but this idea holds promise and might become more common in the future.

● Adductor Tenotomy

The adductor is the muscle that brings the legs together. In some cases during surgery, the doctor needs to make a small cut in a tendon to release this muscle, which is located inside the upper leg near the groin area. This is done so that the tendon can stretch enough for the doctor to put the ball at the top of the thighbone (femoral head) into the right position inside the hip socket. The cut is called an adductor tenotomy, and it can be done together with either a closed reduction or open reduction.

Note: Even though the doctor makes a small cut, this is not the same as an open reduction. In an open reduction the doctor cuts open the hip joint.

Sometimes one or two small stitches are needed to close the tenotomy cut. Usually dissolving stitches are used. Some swelling and bruising are normal in this area. The bruising sometimes does not show until a few days after the surgery and can take a week or two to go away.

Avascular Necrosis (AVN), a Possible Side Effect of Treatment

Avascular necrosis (AVN) is also called osteonecrosis, aseptic necrosis, or ischemic bone necrosis. AVN is a disease in which bone tissue dies because there is not enough blood flow to the bone. AVN in the hip joint can be a complication of treating hip dysplasia in young children.

Over time the reduced blood flow affects the child's bone growth. It also can affect the cartilage near the bone and the joint surface. If the blood supply returns to the area, then the bone tissue can regrow. Regrowth is a slow process that can take many months or up to a year.

During treatment for hip dysplasia, the source of blood to the hip that is most likely to be affected is the medial circumflex femoral artery (MFA). This artery can be stretched and compressed, or compressed between the femoral neck and the labrum (the rim that surrounds the hip joint).

The doctor might need to release a tendon (tenotomy) or shorten the femur (femoral osteotomy) to reduce the risk of AVN. Throughout treatment the doctor monitors your child for this condition. AVN shows up on X rays as white areas. An MRI also can be used to diagnose AVN in its earliest stages which is especially helpful since, in the early stages of AVN, a child may exhibit no obvious symptoms.

Note: If a child has a small femoral head, that does not mean that he or she has AVN. If the whole femoral head is small, it is probably because it is not in correct contact with the hip socket, not because of AVN.

Traction Before Surgery

If a child is from one to three years old when diagnosed with hip dysplasia, then traction might be used before surgery (see Figure 37 on the next page).

During traction, the child's legs are attached with ace bandages and sticky tape to weighted ropes. The ropes go over a frame that is

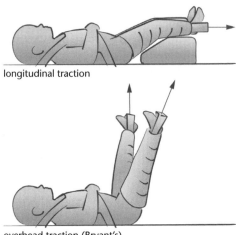

longitudinal traction

overhead traction (Bryant's)

FIGURE 37. A baby in longitudinal traction (top)
and a baby in overhead traction (bottom)

attached to the end of the bed with the weights hanging. The weights are one to two pounds (less than one kilogram) on each side, depending on the size and age of the child. The child stays in traction 24 hours a day with short breaks. This is uncomfortable but not painful.

While your child is in traction, expect him or her to be fussy. Try to find some ways to entertain her while she is lying down:

* Try offering her some small toys.

* Set up a portable DVD player.

* Invite friends and relatives whom she enjoys to visit.

* Cuddle with her. (For this you might have to get creative in your approach. For example, if your child is in traction on the floor, you might have to lie down next to him or her.)

If a child has a condition with muscle contractures, more doctors are inclined to use traction to relax the tight muscles. If the child has flexible muscles and ligaments, then traction is less likely to be needed. Individual doctors have different opinions about how often traction should be used. Traction is more commonly used in some countries than others. In August 2011, the International Hip Dysplasia Institute Medical Advisory Board provided this statement regarding the use of traction:

The place of traction in the treatment of hip dislocations is unclear. It is more widely used in Europe and Asia than in the USA, probably because hospital costs are lower in those countries. It is used in the USA mainly for more severe dislocations. There are two unresolved questions about traction:

1. Does preliminary traction reduce the risk of avascular necrosis (AVN) of the femoral head?

2. Does preliminary traction improve the chances of getting the hip perfectly reduced in the socket?

With regard to AVN, there are some studies that show the hip position in the cast is more important than preliminary traction. There is no evidence that preliminary traction prevents AVN compared to releasing the tendon to take pressure off the femoral head and to allow safer positioning in the cast.

With regard to better chance of reduction, there does seem to be a slightly increased success rate when preliminary traction is used. However, this may benefit more severe dislocations more than minor ones. The tendon release often improves the quality of the reduction.

Currently, in the USA, the most common practice is to do an arthrogram under anesthesia and snip the tendon to help relax the hip (it grows back). If the hip is easily reduced into the socket and can be kept there in a comfortable position, then the cast is used and no traction was needed. On the other hand, when it is difficult to reduce the hip or the position is poor, then there is the choice of using traction for a few weeks before trying the reduction again, or proceeding to a surgical reduction to remove anything that's in the joint and preventing the reduction.

Whether to use traction or not is one of the unsolved questions that the IHDI is attempting to answer with our multi-center trial.

[IHDI MEDICAL BOARD, AUGUST 2011]

Osteotomy Surgery

An osteotomy is surgery in which the doctor cuts bone. Osteotomies for treatment of the hip joint include pelvic osteotomy and femoral osteotomy. A pelvic osteotomy is when the doctor makes one or more cuts in bones in the pelvis, typically near or in the hip socket. A femoral osteotomy is when the doctor makes one or more cuts in the thighbone (femur).

If your child is having an osteotomy, ask the doctor questions to make sure that you understand the treatment. Some questions you might want to ask are listed below:

* Is this a pelvic osteotomy, a femoral osteotomy, or both?
* Can you explain how the osteotomy will help my child?
* Will pins, screws, or plates be needed during this surgery? If so, how long will they be in place?
* If a donor bone will be used, where will you take the donor bone from?
* Will my child limp afterward? If so, for how long?
* Is there anything that my child is not allowed to do while recovering from the osteotomy?

● Pelvic Osteotomy

A pelvic osteotomy is surgery in which the doctor cuts the bone in the pelvis to improve the structure of the hip socket and to improve support for the femoral head. A pelvic osteotomy can be done at the same time as an open reduction. Improvement in the acetabular index (AI) is seen within a year and a half. For more information about the AI, see "Acetabular Index (AI)" on page 24. After a pelvic osteotomy, the child needs strong pain relief medicine for the first two weeks. Make sure that you arrange with the doctor to get the pain relief medicine ahead of time. Sometimes pins are used during the surgery, and they are later removed after the hip has healed.

A pelvic osteotomy is used when other less-invasive methods will not fix the problem. Pelvic osteotomies are usually done for children who are at least three years old, but in some cases, the surgery is done on a child as young as two. Doctors have different opinions about the best age to do this type of surgery. Some will do a pelvic osteotomy together with an open reduction for children as young as 18 months of age. Others wait until children are at least four years old. In children older than four, a pelvic osteotomy can be done to improve the acetabular index (AI). If a closed reduction has already been done, then the doctor waits a year to 18 months to see how the hip socket develops before considering a pelvic osteotomy.

Pelvic osteotomies have many different names, and in some cases the same procedure has more than one name. It is easier to understand this treatment if you think about what kind of improvement the doctor wants to make in the hip-joint structure. Pelvic osteotomies can be loosely grouped into three broad categories, based on the main goal of the surgery. These three categories are volume reducing, positioning, and shelf procedures.

⬤ Volume Reducing Pelvic Osteotomies

This type of surgery reshapes the hip socket and makes it smaller. This surgery is used for younger children when the hip socket is too large. This can happen if the ball at the top of the femur moves in and out of the hip socket and wears it into a large, shallow shape. Examples of this type of surgery are the Pemberton, Dega, and San Diego osteotomies.

Dega Osteotomy. In a Dega osteotomy, a small piece of bone is removed from the top of the pelvis. Then the doctor cuts the bone above the hip socket, tilts it outward, and puts the piece of bone inside.

If the top of the thighbone was up high in the socket (as shown in Figure 38), then that leg might be longer than the other. If this is the case, the doctor can cut the thighbone (do a femoral osteotomy) to equalize the leg lengths.

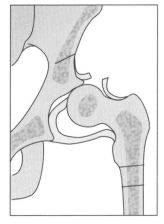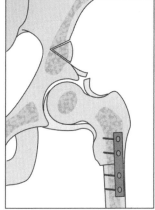

FIGURE 38. A Dega osteotomy

Redirectional Pelvic Osteotomies

This type of osteotomy changes the position of the hip socket. The hip socket is rotated outward into a better position. The procedure that is used depends on the child's age. Typically, a Salter (also called innominate osteotomy) is used for children younger than eight years old. The Steel (also called triple innominate) is used for children between the ages of eight and fifteen years. Periacetabular osteotomy (PAO), which is also called Bernese osteotomy, is used for older teens who have finished growing and for adults.

Salter (Innominate) Osteotomy. A Salter osteotomy (see Figures 39 and 40) can be done together with an open reduction for children from 18 months to six years old. This surgery is often done for children who have bilateral hip dysplasia. The surgeon tilts the acetabulum to correct its angle. The doctor takes a graft of bone from the hip area, cuts through the bone above where the femoral head rests, and inserts the bone graft. One or two 4-inch pins are inserted through all the pieces of bone to hold them together. A typical scar is about 2 inches long.

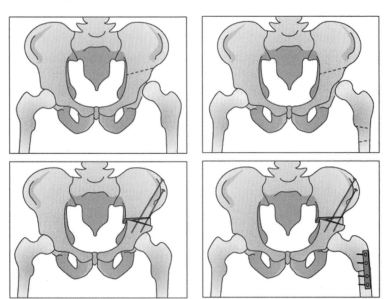

FIGURE 39. A Salter osteotomy

FIGURE 40. A Salter osteotomy combined with a femoral osteotomy

Adolescent Periacetabular Osteotomy (PAO). This surgery is used to create a deeper hip socket with more coverage. A PAO can improve the structure of the hip joint in teens or adults who do not have arthritis and are considered too young to have a total hip replacement (THR). In some cases, a second operation is performed later to remove pins used in the procedure. After healing from the surgery, a PAO will not prevent a woman from having a normal pregnancy. The size of the birth canal remains the same, so the PAO will not cause her to need a cesarean section.

PAO surgery involves a series of steps:

1. The surgeon cuts the bone to allow the top hip socket to move outward (see Figure 41).

2. The doctor rotates the bone outward (see Figure 42).

3. Pins are used to hold the hip joint in place (see Figure 43).

4. As the hip joint heals, new bone grows, making the hip more stable (see Figure 44).

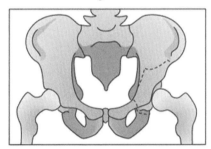

FIGURE 41. PAO surgery. The dotted lines show where the doctor cuts the bone in the pelvis.

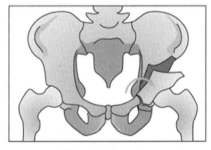

FIGURE 42. When the bone is moved outward, coverage for the hip joint increases.

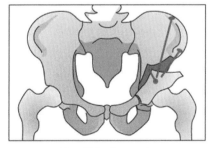

FIGURE 43. The PAO pins are in place.

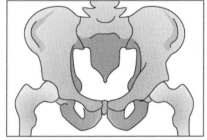

FIGURE 44. After the PAO, the hip joint is more stable.

● Supportive (Shelf Procedure) Pelvic Osteotomies

Shelf procedures add support to the top of the hip socket when the ball at the top of the femur does not have enough coverage. There are a number of different shelf procedures, such as the Albee, Staheli, and Chiari.

Chiari procedure. This can be done for children over four years old, adolescents, or young adults to make the hip socket deeper. The surgeon slides the bone outward to effectively widen the shelf of bone above the femoral head. Steel pins are often used. After the surgery, only partial weight can be put on the leg for three months. This procedure shortens the affected leg. See "Leg-Length Discrepancy" on page 38.

Considerations for Children with Down Syndrome

It is common for children with Down syndrome to develop hip dysplasia. Dr. Charles T. Price, Chairman of the International Hip Dysplasia Institute Medical Board, has this to say about treatment.

Hip dysplasia is more common in Down syndrome than many people realize. We know it gets worse without treatment. Hip instability that occurs in very young children often occurs in the absence of any major changes visible on the X rays. There is a temptation to treat this stage without surgery. Occasional successes have been reported with casts or night bracing, but the condition almost always worsens until surgery is done.

One issue is that the hip tends to dislocate or become dysplastic in a way that is slightly different from standard hip dysplasia. The children with Down syndrome seem to behave more like a traumatic dislocation with a defective posterior wall of the socket. If the child is old enough, it can help greatly to obtain a 3-D CT scan to determine the exact shape of the socket. Femoral osteotomy should be done in addition to any pelvic surgery. The pelvic surgery may consist of a PAO or triple pelvic osteotomy, but "shelf" procedures can be successful when the socket isn't too dysplastic. However, the shelf needs to be a lot more posterior than standard. Recent papers have reported more success with the PAO because the deficiency on the back side of the socket can be corrected more with that procedure.

In the older child who already has changes and erosion visible on the X ray, surgery should be performed as early as possible. The published results of surgery are somewhat discouraging although more current reports using the PAO or triple in younger children have demonstrated improved outcomes. There has been more attention paid to Down syndrome hip dysplasia recently at medical meetings, but there are still few publications with long-term follow-up. Previous surgical attempts have focused on either femoral or pelvic reconstruction with or without tightening of the ligaments around the hips. The more recent recommendations are in line with my personal opinion that surgery should include correction of the posterior deficiency with pelvic and femoral realignment in addition to tightening the ligaments. When all three things are done, there is probably a better chance of correcting the problem.

My thoughts in summary are as follows: Surgery is almost the only way to stop it from getting worse. Combined procedures seem to work better than only correcting one component even when the other components seem to be normal in shape. It's probably best to overcorrect beyond the normal shape to keep the hip from dislocating again. Finally, the results of successful surgery are much better than doing nothing and watching the hip deteriorate. Kids with Down syndrome don't complain of pain much, but this can become pretty disabling when left alone.   [CHARLES T. PRICE, MD]

Arthroscopy to Repair a Torn Labrum (Adolescent)

The labrum is the soft rim of cartilage that surrounds the hip joint. Hip dysplasia can be associated with labrums that are larger than usual. The enlarged labrum provides some support to the joint when the hip socket is shallow. But in some teens and adults, the labrum

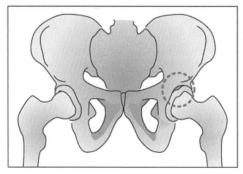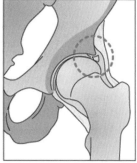

FIGURE 45. A hip joint with a torn labrum

develops a tear because of the stress on it from the shallow hip socket (see Figure 45). A labral tear is painful and sometimes leads to a diagnosis of previously undetected hip dysplasia in a teen or young adult.

Labral tears can be repaired arthroscopically at the same time an osteotomy is done to improve the alignment of the bones in the hip joint. During an arthroscopy, the doctor uses a surgical tool called an arthroscope, which is about the size of a pencil, to examine the cartilage. Depending on the condition of the labrum, the doctor might stitch torn cartilage, trim it, or remove loose pieces. For hospitals with large hip centers, two doctors might work together as a team in which one doctor does the osteotomy and one repairs the labrum.

For people who do not have hip dysplasia, labral tears caused by sports injuries can sometimes be repaired using only arthroscopy surgery. However, for people with both hip dysplasia and a labral tear, arthroscopy alone does not solve the underlying problem that caused the tear and can actually make the hip less stable. The reason for this is that the underlying bone structure of the hip joint led to the labral tear, and trimming the labrum removes the extra support that the labrum had been providing.

Femoral Osteotomy

A femoral osteotomy is surgery in which the doctor cuts the thighbone (femur). This can be done to correct a leg-length discrepancy (one leg is much longer than the other) or to correct the angle at which the ball at the top of the femur (femoral head) meets the hip socket. A femoral osteotomy that corrects this angle is called a varus derotational osteotomy (VDO or VDRO). *Varus* means "inward," so in this procedure, the femoral head is tilted inward toward the center of the body. For children under four years of age, this surgery might be done to treat acetabular dysplasia.

Figure 46 shows how the angles differ between the left and right hips before a VDO.

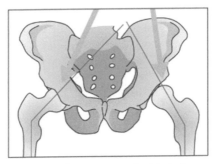

FIGURE 46. The structure of a hip before a varus derotational femoral osteotomy

After the surgery, the angle of the hip shown on the right has improved (see Figure 47). A plate and screws are used to secure the femur until it has healed.

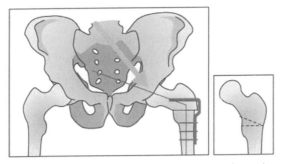

FIGURE 47. The structure of a hip after a varus derotational femoral osteotomy

After this surgery, a child up to about age six wears a spica cast for up to eight weeks to hold the hip joint in position. Older children and adolescents who are not wearing a cast might have movement restrictions such as not being allowed to cross their legs. For children who are still growing, the plate and screws are removed later in a separate operation.

A VDO corrects the angle at which the femoral head meets the hip socket. If a child's hip is dislocated and the femoral head is up above the hip socket in a high dislocation, the affected leg often has grown longer than the other leg to compensate for this position. If this is the case, when the doctor does the femoral osteotomy, he or she can remove some extra length from the top of the femur. This makes it easier for the femoral head to go inside the hip socket in the correct alignment without stretching the entire leg and potentially damaging the surrounding soft tissue (muscles, ligaments, nerves and so on). After the surgery if the child's operated leg is shorter, it typically grows longer so that the leg lengths equalize.

A femoral osteotomy can be done together with an open reduction or a pelvic osteotomy. The type of surgery depends on the structure of the hip joint and the age of the child.

Removing Pins or a Plate and Screws after an Osteotomy

If a young child's surgery required pins, or a metal plate and screws, he or she will need another surgery to remove them after the bone has healed to prevent the bone from growing over them and covering them. If bone covers the pins or plate and screws, this makes any future surgeries difficult, even a surgery in later life such as a total hip replacement when a person is in his or her seventies. The length of time for the bone to heal after a child's surgery can range from eight weeks after a pelvic osteotomy to one year after a femoral osteotomy, but the surgery to remove pins or plates and screws can be done up to three years after the osteotomy. After three years, the surgery is more difficult.

Usually removing pins or a plate and screws is a fairly quick surgery; often the child goes home afterward without staying overnight at the hospital. Your child will be sore for a few days and probably will need pain relief. He or she might not want to move much. In some cases, the doctor limits the child's activities during recovery. For example, the child might need to stay off his or her feet for a week or two after the surgery. Pins or plates and screws are removed for teens if they are still growing or if the pins bother them after the bone has healed.

Total Hip Replacement (THR)

It is very rare for a teen to need hip joint replacement, but it does happen. Hip joint replacement is also called total hip replacement (THR) and total hip arthroplasty (THA). Hip resurfacing, a surgery that uses a different kind of implants, is not usually recommended for adolescents or adults with hip dysplasia.[3]

Generally, the decision for a young person to have a THR would only happen if other less-invasive treatments have not worked. THR might be used to treat adolescents when all of the following conditions apply:

* The teen or young adult is in chronic pain, the hip joint is deteriorating, and it has not responded to less-invasive treatment.

* The hip-joint structure is not congruent, which means that PAO surgery is not recommended. The shape of the hip socket and the ball at the top of the femur prevent them from fitting together in a healthy alignment.

* The teen or young adult has finished growing or is nearly finished growing.

During THR surgery, the femoral head is replaced with an implant in the shape of a ball with a stem, and a corresponding cup-shaped implant is inserted into the hip socket. There are many types of implants, and they can be made of different materials such as metal, metal and plastic, or ceramic. Figure 48 on the next page shows an X ray of a hip after surgery. The implants show up as white shapes.

Depending on the shape of the hip joint, special implants are sometimes needed for people who have hip dysplasia. The doctor selects the implant and can explain the reasons for his or her choice to you.

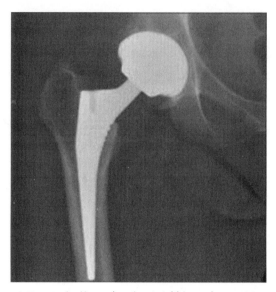

FIGURE 48. An X ray showing total hip replacement (THR) implants

The doctor might recommend preoperative exercises. Many hospitals offer a class in which patients can learn about THR surgery. For more information about THR surgery in connection with hip dysplasia, see the International Hip Dysplasia Institute website www.hipdysplasia.org and the book *A Guide for Adults with Hip Dysplasia* (West and Sutherland).

Adult Treatment

Early treatment for hip dysplasia is typically quite effective. As one parent of a baby with hip dysplasia said:

> I had [hip dysplasia] myself as a baby. I was in the Pavlik harness from birth until two months of age, and then in a night brace until I was six months old. I have never had any residual hip issues and never would have known I ever had anything wrong with me had I not talked to my mom.   **[MEGAN]**

Most cases of hip dysplasia are resolved like Megan's. However, if you were treated for hip dysplasia in infancy or childhood, and your case was difficult or you were diagnosed late, you could have some residual hip dysplasia. This means that treatment improved your hip structure but did not completely correct the problem. Some people are not diagnosed with hip dysplasia until adulthood. For instance, the Olympic gold medalist Mary Lou Retton had undiagnosed hip dysplasia, which caused her to need total hip replacement surgery when she was in her thirties.

If you are an adult and think you might have undiagnosed hip dysplasia, see your doctor. If it turns out that you have residual hip dysplasia or are diagnosed with untreated hip dysplasia, your orthopedic doctor develops a treatment plan based on your individual case. Hip dysplasia can range from mild to severe. If you have mild symptoms, your doctor can probably help you manage them without surgery. Some common nonsurgical treatments for adults with hip dysplasia are listed below.

● Pain Relief

Typically nonsteroidal anti-inflammatory drugs (NSAIDs) such as ibuprofen are used to relieve pain and reduce inflammation in the hip joints. Your doctor recommends the type of medicine and the correct dosage.

● Exams and X Rays to Monitor Joint Health

Your orthopedic doctor might want to examine your hips and see X rays of your hips at specific intervals, such as every two years.

You could discover that making some changes in your daily life helps your hips feel better. For instance, you might not be able to tolerate standing or walking on hard surfaces for extended periods of time. Some other suggestions are listed here:

Exercise and Weight Management

It is important to stay active and maintain a healthy weight because gaining weight tends to stress the hip joints, which can increase hip pain. Ask your orthopedic doctor which types of exercise would be best for you and whether there is anything you should not do. This might change as you get older. For example, up until middle age, I did not have any restrictions, but now my orthopedic doctor advises me to avoid running and other high-impact exercises.

A Comfortable Mattress
If your hips bother you at night, consider trying a different mattress, such as a pillowtop or a Memory Foam mattress cover.

Are Your Hips Sensitive to Hormonal Changes?
For some women with hip dysplasia, their hips improve or feel worse, depending on whether they are pregnant, taking birth control pills, or experiencing a menstrual cycle. This is highly individual consideration and does not apply in every case. If you think hormonal changes are aggravating your hip dysplasia, bring it up with your orthopedic doctor.

If You Are Experiencing Chronic, Severe Pain, Your Doctor Might Recommend Surgery

When your doctor recommends surgery for your hip dysplasia, the type of surgery depends on your age, your hip-joint structure, and whether you have osteoarthritis in your hip joints, as well as your pain level and quality of life (how well you can manage daily tasks). The main surgeries to treat hip dysplasia in adult are periacetabular osteotomy (PAO) and total hip replacement (THR).

For more information about adult treatment, see the International Hip Dysplasia Institute website www.hipdysplasia.org and the book *A Guide for Adults with Hip Dysplasia* (West and Sutherland).

Optional Physical Therapy Exercises Before a PAO

Being healthy and fit before surgery helps you tolerate the surgery and improves the healing and recovery process. Physical therapy (PT) before a PAO is not commonly prescribed, but it can be used to help reduce some symptoms by improving hip stability, strength, flexibility, and balance, and to aid in recovery by building muscle memory. Muscle memory means that if you repeat a movement pattern or exercise, then your body is more likely to remember and repeat the same movement in the future, such as during physical therapy exercises that come after surgery.

The PT program depends on the activity level of the individual and his or her age. These exercises are optional and are meant for adults who can do them without pain. Teens could potentially benefit as well, based on the guidance of the doctor and physical therapist. Ask your orthopedic doctor about seeing a physical therapist and which types of exercise would be best for you. It is also important to know if the doctor recommends that you avoid any particular activities or exercises.

The goals of pre-op PT are to:

* Manage current symptoms.

* Maintain function and prevent compensatory gait patterns (limping).

* Prevent wear and tear of the hip joint and cartilage.

* Prepare the body for surgery.

* Provide a "preview" of post-op physical therapy.

* Encourage muscle memory to prevent post-op atrophy (the tendency for muscles to lose strength over time when they are not used).

All exercises should be pain free. If you experiences pain, stop the exercise and contact the physical therapist about modifying the exercise or trying a different one. The following exercises are examples of the types of movements that might be recommended.

* Stand and squeeze the buttocks of one leg (keeping hip stable) while lifting the opposite knee toward your chest. This exercise stabilizes and strengthens the hip.

* On your hands and knees, rock back and forth within a pain-free zone. This lubricates the hip joint with synovial fluid and maintains range of motion.

* On your hands and knees, do hip extensions into leg lifts. This strengthens the gluteal muscles that stabilize the hip joint.

* Psoas strengthening. The psoas is the muscle that connects the lower portion of your back to the top of your thigh. It is a muscle

important to your core strength, so it is important to keep it strong. For the exercise, sit in a chair with your back straight. Raise one thigh toward your chest. You can apply gentle downward pressure on your knee with your hands to increase the challenge.

* Lie on your side and do straight leg raises. This exercise strengthens the outer hip and gluteal muscles.

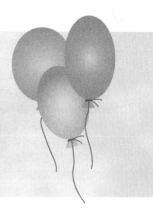

8

Caring for a
Child in a Cast

After a reduction or osteotomy, babies and young children wear spica casts or Petrie casts (also called Bachelor casts) to keep the hips in the correct position. Both types of casts are described in this chapter. The child usually wears the cast from twelve to twenty weeks after a reduction. The length of time in a cast after an osteotomy is usually shorter. Because children grow quickly, each child usually needs a cast change at least once during treatment. The cast is removed, and a new one is put on. Often the new cast is less restrictive than the first one. For example, the first cast might come to a child's ankles, and the second cast might come to the child's knees. Expect your child to take a week to ten days to recover from surgery and adjust to the cast.

When a baby or young child is put into a cast, it is harder to snuggle up together, but it is still worth the effort. Nursing mothers can continue to breast-feed a baby in a cast. Take the time to find ways to get skin-to-skin contact with your baby or child. Tickle his or her chin, hold hands, or stroke his or her hair. As one mother says:

The funny thing is that before the surgery she wasn't very cuddly, but now she does her best to lay her head on our shoulder or chest and uses her hands to pull us toward her, so I know she needs that as much as we do. It's very hard to get past the cast and remember she's a real baby in there. It seems so unhuman, but then you look at her sweet face, and you know she's a little baby, like all the others. It helps to take off all her clothes and peer down into the cast and see her sweet tummy and belly button and her soft little back. It helps to make her seem real and normal. **[HIP-BABY DISCUSSION GROUP]**

Spica Cast

A spica cast is a body cast that covers the pelvis and holds the hip joints in place (see Figure 49).

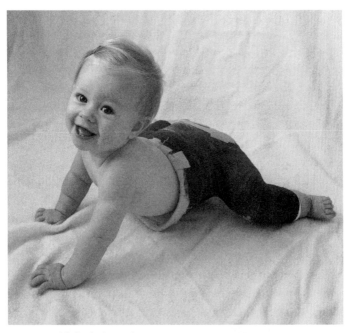

FIGURE 49. Violet in her spica cast *(Photo courtesy of Jesi Josten)*

A spica cast has an outer layer that can be made of plaster or fiberglass and an inner lining that can be made of cotton or Gore-Tex (a water-resistant fabric). A plaster cast must be kept dry so that it stays hard and firm to hold the hips in place. Cotton lining should also be kept dry. Many parents like the combination of fiberglass and Gore-

Tex because the cast can get wet without being damaged, and the child can take a bath or shower. See "Bathing a Child in a Fiberglass and Gore-Tex Cast" on page 131. However, some children's hands become red and irritated from touching the fiberglass. Some doctors prefer cotton lining because it can be packed more firmly and can lessen the chance of skin irritation. Cotton is softer and provides more of a cushion between the child and the cast. Ask for your doctor's preference and the reason for it.

Petrie Cast (Also Called a Bachelor Cast)

This cast is more common in Australia than in the United States. In the United States, it is sometimes used when a cast is changed after the spica. It works like a brace, with the legs in the cast but not the pelvis. A bar like a broomstick connects the legs of the cast (see Figure 50).

Children can learn to sit up in this type of cast, and you might be able to use normal diapers. To lift a child in this cast, support the

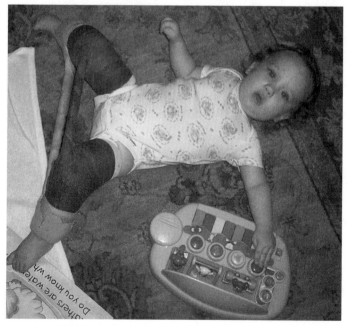

FIGURE 50. Addison in her Petrie cast *(Photo courtesy of Elle Pampinella)*

child's bottom and weight. Do not try to use the bar to lift up the child. Some parents attach toys to the bar when a baby is sitting up and playing. Then if he or she drops them, they are easy to retrieve.

When you have an older child who will be wearing a cast, plan to purchase extra pillows and pillowcases. Consider using a wedge pillow to prop up your child's head. Figure 51 shows Megan in her cast. (Note the row of dollar bills with notes on them attached to the wall. Megan's grandparents sent her a dollar and a note every week that she was wearing the cast.)

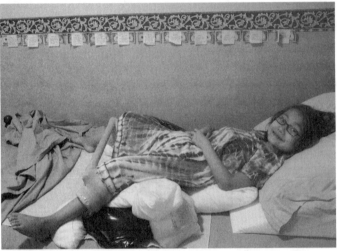

FIGURE 51. Megan, age seven, looking comfy in her Petrie cast. Note the wedge pillow and other cushions. *(Photo courtesy of Patti Sheeter)*

Getting Used to the Cast

As much as possible, treat your child as you usually do. He will sense your attitude and react to it. Of course you should respond if your child is in pain or needs help but do not feel as if you have to jump every time he makes a sound. Give your child a little time to settle, just as you would with any other child or new situation. Set him up to eat at the table with the rest of the family at mealtimes.

Patti Streeter offers this advice based on her experience when her daughter, Megan (seven years old), was in a spica cast:

Experiment! We found as we got more used to the cast, we weren't as nervous to try new things. We figured out how to prop her in a folding chair, which then allowed her to eat at the table much easier and use the computer. We had her on the floor. We had her in our bed. You really can't hurt the kids when they're in the cast. They do need support around the cast, and you have to watch you aren't creating any pressure places (like around the leg openings). But don't be afraid to try new positions, locations, etc.   **[PATTI]**

At first the idea of caring for a child in a cast may seem like running a slow-motion marathon. Everything takes longer than it ought to and facing the weeks or months of treatment ahead is daunting. As you and your child develop routines, life with the cast becomes easier to manage.

Remember that in spite of the fact that your child's hips are the center of your universe now, this will not always be the case. There is far more to your child than his hips and far more to you than being his caretaker, as important a job as that is. Take the time to appreciate the good moments with your child, and there will be good moments, though at first this could be hard to believe.

One mother calls her daughter Delaney her "3-foot hero." Delaney, who has an unusually severe case of hip dysplasia, has been through many surgeries:

Delaney has taught me so much... To slow down and enjoy things in "baby steps." PATIENCE, PATIENCE, and more PATIENCE! The actual meaning of strength and perseverance—not the textbook version. That heroes can be three feet tall! That I am stronger than I thought. That I can make the tough decisions and follow through with them. That a smile CAN light up a room. That one person, no matter how small, can impact a lot of lives. I am sure there are lots more. What has your hip baby taught you?   **[HEATHER]**

Don't be afraid to ask for help or to accept help from others. When Vivian's daughter, Angela, had surgery, one of the mothers at school had this creative idea about how to help.

Last year, one of the moms of a little girl in Angela's kindergarten class organized it so every day one of her classmates would visit with an activity and they brought a meal for our family. This was EX-TREMELY helpful since it helped us out in many ways. It kept Angela busy, she got to visit with a different classmate every day which kept her connected to her class, the parents sat with her so I could run out and do errands, and I had I didn't have to worry about dinner for my family. I also received many gift cards for restaurants from our friends to help with meals.

Having people help with meals and sit with my kids while I did errands was most helpful. I'm a stay-at-home mom, and my husband travels a lot for work. It was very difficult to handle all my kids and Angela in her cast. I wouldn't have been able to do it without all the help from my friends and family.   [VIVIAN]

Comforting a Fussy Child

Kiera had an open reduction with bilateral pelvic osteotomies at age two and a half. Her mother describes Kiera's adjustment to being in the cast in the following quote:

She was old enough to know that she used to be able to walk and run around, old enough to know that she could no longer move with the cast on, old enough to verbalize the fact that she didn't like it, but NOT old enough to understand why we were putting her through this. A bad combination, but after the five or six days, during which she was angry, depressed, in pain, and scared, she bounced back and was her normal, cheerful, funny self. Of course, she was still a toddler with tantrums...but I digress.   [LAURIE]

It can be hard to tell if a child is fussy because of a problem with the cast or as a result of something else such as teething, an ear infection, or some other ailment. Here are some things to try:

* Change her diaper. During the diaper change, check for any skin irritation or diaper rash.

* Some babies spit up more in a cast. If this is the case, check with your pediatrician about the best medicine to reduce the problem.

* If the weather is hot and your child is in a cast, do what you can to cool her off. If the cast is waterproof, let her play in the water. If the cast cannot get wet, dress your child in as little as possible and sponge off her skin with a damp cloth. Or fill up the sink with water and sit with the child in your lap. Let your child reach in and splash the water with a towel over her lap.

Moving or Lifting a Child in a Cast

When you lift your child, use care. The cast adds about five pounds, but it feels like more because when you pick up your child, he or she can't move in response. It can take practice to get used to it. Here are some suggestions:

* If your child's cast has a bar between the legs, do not use the bar to lift the cast. This can damage the cast and could possibly affect the position of your child's hips. Protect your back by using safe lifting techniques. Bend your knees and place one arm beneath your child's shoulders and your other arm beneath his buttocks. If two people are lifting him, one person supports his shoulders while the other lifts his legs.

* Vary your child's position during the day and move him into different rooms in the house. You can use a stroller or a wagon with pillows to make this easier. An older child can use a reclining wheelchair.

* When settling your child onto a flat surface, use rolled-up towels or small pillows to support his feet or legs. Make sure that your child is comfortable and the edges of the cast do not press against his skin. For example, when a child is on his stomach, place rolled-up towels beneath the front of his ankles to support them.

Cast Care

Inspect the inside of the cast daily. You can use a flashlight to check for small objects that can irritate the skin such as crumbs or dry cereal. Often the edges of the cast have waterproof tape applied. This is sometimes called petalling the cast.

● Taping the Edges of the Cast (Petalling)

You can apply waterproof tape to the edges of the cast to help keep it clean. This is called petalling because of the way the tape looks. Petalling makes a smoother surface against your child's skin than the cast. It also adds a barrier in case urine or stool leaks out of the diaper. If the tape gets soiled, it can be removed and replaced with clean tape. Over time, the tape tends to come off the chest area. Some recommended tapes are listed here:

* Nexcare waterproof tape, which is available at Walmart and Target stores

* Hy-tape, which is pink and sometimes used at hospitals for wound care, or tegaderm hospital tape

* Moleskin, which is sold in drugstores alongside the Dr. Scholl's items (add more layers rather than trying to pull off the old tape)

To apply the waterproof tape:

1. Cut 4-inch (10 cm) lengths of tape.

2. Wrap a piece of tape over the edge of the cast.

3. Add another piece right next to it, overlapping as you go. Work your way all around the opening of the cast.

Note: Some parents line the cast opening with panty liners to protect the tape. Tape them in place with medical tape.

● Cast Odors

No matter how careful you are when you change your baby, the cast probably will get soiled. To help with odors, you can try these ideas:

* Use a blow-dryer on a cool setting to dry out a wet lining. A product called the CastCooler can also help remove moisture from a cast. See the Resources section of this book on page 188.

* Apply an odor eliminator or perfume to the cast (not on the child). Use it sparingly to avoid getting the cast damp or interfering with the normal airflow through the cast.

* Remove any old or dirty bandage material from inside the cast.

* Completely change all the tape.

When cleaning up your child, don't be afraid to put your hands inside the cast. You might be able to put a cloth down the front of the cast over the stomach and pull it out the diaper area.

Diapering

If possible, ask a nurse to help you practice changing a diaper at the hospital before you take your child home. Change the diaper regularly to prevent any wetness from the diaper from wicking into the cast. Remove the inner diaper slowly from the front first, so that you can prevent stool from touching the cast when the diaper is removed.

For some babies, the small diaper isn't needed—an incontinence pad inside the cast with a large diaper fastened outside is enough. Try both methods to see which works best for you. Some parents use a combination of incontinence pads, maxi pads, and diapers. The following are good supplies to have on hand:

* small disposable diapers (size 1)

* large disposable diapers (size 5)

* adult incontinence pads (such as Poise Ultra with side shields, or the CVS brand)

* 12-inch (30 cm) lengths of cotton from a cotton roll (this is sometimes used by hair stylists for perms)

* tongue depressors or Popsicle sticks (sold at craft stores)

* baby powder and a barrier cream such as Neosporin

Tip: For a boy, incontinence pads might not work because he needs more room in the front, and the pad in front can get too full too fast. Try a diaper that is wide in the crotch area such as Pampers Swaddlers New Baby. If you use Pampers diapers, make sure that the cartoon character cannot be seen on the front side. For Huggies brand diapers, make sure the character is centered over his penis.

● *How to Change a Disposable Diaper*

You might want to tape the edges of the cast to keep it clean before you remove a diaper for the first time. See "Taping the Edges of the Cast (Petalling)" on page 128. The following are step-by-step instructions for how to change a disposable diaper:

1. Tear or cut off the tapes on the back of the size-1 diaper. Do not cut off the elastic. It helps the diaper hold its shape.

   Tip: The size-1 diaper should be oval. If you cut off too much and the diaper gets soaked, the absorbent material can bead up and out the sides of the diaper and into the cast.

2. For extra protection, you can use an incontinence pad and cotton strips.

   Tips: Center the incontinence pad inside the size-1 diaper and press down to stick it in place. Fold 12-inch (30 cm) cotton strips in half and tuck them around the baby's legs, just inside the edge of the cast. You can also tuck cotton strips inside the legs of the cast and up the back. During diaper changes, carefully pull the strips back up and replace them the next time.

3. Lift the baby's buttocks and slip the small diaper into the back of the cast.

   Tips: You can use a tongue depressor or Popsicle stick to help tuck in the diaper. Baby powder on the child's bottom helps the diaper slip over the baby's skin. You might find it easier to turn your child over onto his or her tummy and push the diaper up into the cast. Then lay the child on his or her back for the next step.

4. Pull the diaper up (under the bar for a Petrie cast) and tuck it into the front.

   Tip: If you are diapering a boy, his penis should be pointing up, not down.

5. Put the size-5 diaper on outside of the cast.

● *How to Change a Cloth Diaper*

These instructions are for prefolded cloth diapers and a cast with a Gore-Tex liner. You can use newborn size or diaper inserts (the kind that look like disposables with Velcro tabs). You will need a diaper and a waterproof diaper cover.

1. Fold a prefold into thirds. If there are tabs, fold them inside.

2. Start with the front. Hold the diaper with the folded side out to prevent chafing. Tuck in a little at first. Then slide it up and keep tucking around the cast sides and back.

3. Tuck in the back and pull out a little from the front for a "poop pouch." It doesn't need to look pretty to work.

4. Put on a waterproof cover to keep clothes dry.

Toileting

If your child is old enough to use the toilet, you can try a bedpan, or if the child is tall enough, help him or her stand next to or over the toilet. If the cast lets the child bend at the waist, you can have him or her sit backward on the toilet seat facing the tank. For girls a female urinal can be used instead of a bedpan. Steps Charity has made a series of videos about caring for children in spica casts, including one about toileting. See "Online Video Resources" in the "Resources" section on page 189 for the link. To let a child wear underwear, some families have bought underwear in a much larger size and then sewed Velcro or ties onto the sides so that it can be fastened on top of the cast.

Washing Up

You will need to make some adjustments to your routine. If your child is wearing a plaster cast, it must be kept dry, which means that baths or showers are not allowed. The following sections offer some suggestions to help with your child's personal hygiene.

● Bathing a Child in a Fiberglass and Gore-Tex Cast

If your child is wearing a fiberglass cast with Gore-Tex lining, you can bathe him, cast and all. You might find it works best to get into the bath or shower with your child.

The cast dries faster after a shower than a bath. That is something to consider, depending on the weather. If it is very warm, using the bath will help your child stay cool as the cast slowly dries out. In winter, a shower is a better idea. To use the shower, one parent can get into the shower and hold the child. The other parent then gently rinses out the cast. When bathing a child in the bathtub, a parent can get into the bathtub, with the child sitting on the adult's legs. Some doctors limit the number of baths allowed per week while a child is in a cast.

When the cast is wet, it takes about two hours to dry out on a hot day. The water that gets inside the cast turns to vapor from the warmth of the child's body. Then it passes through the Gore-Tex lining and the cast. You also can dry the cast with a blow dryer set on low. This takes 45 to 60 minutes. Your child's clothes will be damp until the cast is dry.

● Skin Care

Skin irritation is common when children wear a cast. One place to check is the creases of the child's thighs. If the skin is irritated, clean it gently with a soft washcloth and apply a diaper cream such as Balmex or Neosporin. If the child's skin becomes very irritated where the edge of the cast rubs, try using panty liners around the edge. Or you can put cheesecloth (available at grocery stores) through the cast to form a barrier and treat the rash with Desitin ointment. Remove the cheesecloth later to keep the cast from absorbing the Desitin ointment. Also see "Taping the Edges of the Cast (Petalling)" on page 128.

Incisions

An incision is the place where the doctor made a cut for an open reduction or osteotomy. If your child has an incision, it will not develop a scab. This is normal. Signs of infection include redness, tenderness, swelling, and fever. If you are concerned about the incision, contact your doctor. In many cases, the incision is covered by the cast and cannot be seen. The incision usually heals within two weeks. Your child's doctor will give you instructions about what to look for concerning any potential problems with the incision while it is healing.

The appearance of the incision scar depends on the child's skin type and the kind of surgery. For an open reduction or pelvic osteotomy, the scar is located in the groin area and is about 2 to 3 inches (5 to 7.5 cm) long. When healed, this scar typically looks like a crease in the skin. A femoral osteotomy scar on the thigh will increase in length as the child grows. It can take up to a year for a scar to take on its final appearance. If plates and screws from an osteotomy need to be removed later (up to a year after the first surgery), the doctor usually reopens the original scar to avoid creating a new one.

Sores

Though most children have only minor skin irritation, it is helpful to know how to treat a sore if one develops. For a painful sore that does not have a scab, ask your pharmacist about a hydrocolloidal bandage. This is a special kind of bandage made for open sores or burns.

● *Hair Care*

If your child is in a plaster spica cast, you can lay her on the kitchen counter and wash her hair over the sink. If this doesn't work, try a shampoo cap or a dry shampoo such as Johnson's Kids "No More Bedhead." Also, try braids for longer hair.

Clothing Tips

While your child is in a cast, try these tips to make dressing as easy—and as comfortable for your child—as possible:

* Buy clothes a size or two larger than your child would normally wear.

* Use footed pajamas and leave open some of the snaps.

* Try T-shirts, pullovers, or kimono style shirts. When it is cold, sweatshirts will also work.

* Use Add-a-Size garment extenders available through One Step Ahead on onesies. This will make the leg openings bigger.

* Take advantage of loose dresses. Some people will assume that your little girl is wearing tights rather than a cast.

* Try overalls. Overalls that snap all the way to the ankle might fit over the cast, depending on the angle of the child's legs.

Breast-Feeding

Moms who are breast-feeding can continue to do so while the child is in a cast. As one woman said in response to a new mom's anxiety:

You can definitely breast-feed in a spica cast, and, no, it isn't all that difficult. It sounds hard, and it does take a bit of practice in the beginning, but once you get the hang of it, it's no big deal. I nursed my daughter through two spicas, one from four to seven months and another from eleven months to thirteen months, and she's still going strong at eighteen months. **[HIP-BABY DISCUSSION GROUP]**

When breast-feeding, positioning is important, and it can be tricky because with the cast on, your baby does not curve around your body. Try to find a position in which your baby doesn't have to turn her head very much to latch on. The following advice comes from women who have direct experience. Here are some methods that worked for them:

* Lay your baby across your lap as usual. You can put a pillow under her if it helps. Depending on the angle of the cast, one leg might be up in the air close to your shoulder. If that is the case, put your arm between the baby's legs to support him or her.

* While you are sitting, cross one leg over the other to position the baby near your breast (see Figure 52). Your baby will have to turn

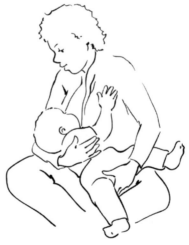

FIGURE 52. A mother breast-feeding a child in a spica cast

her head to latch on. Your baby might latch on at the wrong angle, which is painful. If this happens, take the baby off the breast, reposition, and try again.

* Have your baby straddle one of your legs. Then tip her to the side to nurse from the opposite breast. This upright position (see Figure 53) can be good for a child who spits up or has reflux. If the cast rubs against your leg, put a small pillow on your thigh under the baby. This can work well for a young baby. Some mothers prefer this position when nursing in public.

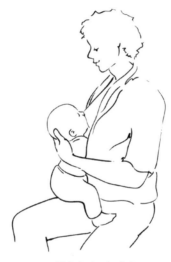

FIGURE 53. This baby is sitting up
while breast-feeding in a spica cast.

* Breast-feed your baby in bed. If you turn slightly to the side, this can make it easier for your baby to latch on. Prop a pillow behind your baby to position him or her. You can move the pillow and put the baby on his or her back when you're done. You can also put the pillow under his or her legs to support them. Make sure that you are toward the middle of the bed so that you don't have to worry about your baby being too close to the edge. You can also try a semireclined position. Lie on your back either in bed with a couple of pillows for support or in a recliner. Put the baby on your stomach and chest.

Eating and Nutrition

Many children eat less while they are wearing a cast. Because they are less active, they might not be as hungry as before. It is common for a child to gain very little weight while wearing a cast.

Some children spit up more often when they wear a cast. This can be due to the cast pressing against a child's stomach when he leans forward. If your child is eating and drinking well and is not bothered by spitting up, then this is not a cause for worry. If your child spits up frequently, seems distressed, or has a history of gastric reflux (GERD), work with your pediatrician's office. Depending on the kind of cast the child is wearing, it is sometimes possible to cut a window in the front to allow more room for his stomach to expand after eating. If your child is already taking medicine for GERD, your doctor might need to adjust the dosage.

Some children have trouble with constipation when wearing a cast. When a child is constipated, she has hard stools that could be painful to pass. This might be because she is moving less than usual due to the restriction of the cast. If this is the case, check with your pediatrician's office for suggestions about how to reduce the constipation. Some common drinks and foods that can help your child to be more regular are fruits, fruit juices, vegetables, and whole grains. Other foods, such as rice can contribute to constipation. Your pediatrician's office should have a list of foods that help relieve constipation, as well as foods to avoid. Many parenting books also include this information. Some children find it easier to have a bowel movement when they are lying on their stomachs.

Rolling Over, Crawling, or Standing

Your pediatric orthopedic doctor will explain any restrictions your child might have. Some children should not crawl, stand, or walk while wearing a cast. This depends on your child's individual circumstances. Many children figure out how to roll over from back to front, or from front to back. Some scoot on the floor, crawl, or even pull up and walk (see Figure 54). Your child's upper body could become very strong from moving with the cast on.

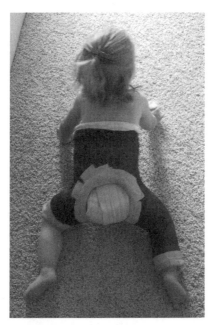

FIGURE 54. Violet crawling, wearing her cast *(Photo courtesy of Jesi Josten)*

At the same time, your child's abdominal muscles and lower body lose muscle tone during treatment with the cast. This is normal, and after the cast is removed, your child will gradually regain muscle tone in those areas.

Delaney had bilateral open reductions with femoral osteotomies when she was 18 months old. Being in a cast did not slow her down.

Delaney would crawl all over the place in [the cast]. She wore out the knees of it in six weeks. She could roll over, turn, and back up.

Don't think that a spica will slow these kids down much. My daughter also has cerebral palsy that affects her leg, left side more than right, and also affects her arms. She managed just fine in a spica. Like I said, she crawled everywhere. By the time she came out of it, she had the most toned little arms you have ever seen.

[HEATHER]

Some children wear out the knees of a cast from crawling. If your child crawls, check his or her legs where the edges of the cast are to make sure the skin does not get irritated. You can put adult socks over the knees to prevent holes in clothing from crawling in a cast. If your doctor allows your child to cruise in a cast, he or she might like an empty laundry basket that is turned upside-down. The child can use it for a little extra support, and push it around like a walker.

Play Time

Here are some ideas for passing the time:

* Prop up your child on the floor with a bed-rest pillow. Then place a breakfast-in-bed tray table in front of him with toys on it.
* Watch videos that encourage movement, such as *The Wiggles*. Encourage your child to "dance" with his upper body.
* Provide small toys such as little people and blocks, or a Lego table with Lego or Duplo blocks.
* Offer simple art supplies such as coloring books, crayons, stickers, or pipe cleaners to keep your child occupied. An easel can also be fun. Put the child in a stroller placed next to the easel.
* Provide fun manipulatives, such as counting bears and pattern blocks.
* Sit your child on your lap and play on the computer.
* Read together.
* Get out of the house every day. Go for a walk.
* Blow bubbles or use a toy that makes bubbles when turned on.
* Schedule play dates for him. Invite friends and family to visit.
* Give him some down time. Set him up with toys in a safe area and do something in another room, such as making dinner in the kitchen.
* Put large pasta noodles or dried beans in a cake pan or container and give the child measuring cups and spoons.
* Buy or make Play-Doh.
* Try magnetic storyboards, Magnadoodle, or aquadoodle mini mats.

Adapting Your Home
for a Child in a Cast

Patti Sheeter's daughter Megan was seven when she had surgery for hip dysplasia, and she wore a cast afterward. Patti offers these suggestions for parents of older children who wear spica casts after surgery for hip dysplasia:

* You will want a reclining wheelchair. Have the hospital fit your child for the wheelchair after the surgery! Our loaner chair was delivered to us while Megan was in surgery, and it turned out to be too narrow for the cast.

* Ask about Z-Flow Positioners while you are inpatient. Our hospital used them in-patient, and then we were allowed to bring them home with us. They are great! They are moldable pillows. Think Play-Doh in a Ziploc bag. They come in three or four sizes, and we used them to position Megan in bed, on the couch, etc.

* You might want to look into a wedge pillow, too. That has been great for sleeping and for belly time. We had to have a prescription for it, but we were then able to pick it up from a local home health supply store.

* Buy lots of extra pillowcases! We had six sets (two pillowcases each set) that we rotated. They [children in treatment] spend a lot of time propped in bed or on the couch with pillows, so it is nice to be able to switch them out often. Extra pillows are good, too. We used two pillows on the reclining wheelchair—one on the seat, and one on the back—to add support and make it a bit more comfortable. We also bought some new, fun bed sheets. Since Megan was going to be in her bed so much, we tried to make it a little exciting.

⬤ *Furniture*

Chairs can be a challenge, especially for a child in a cast. The angle of the cast varies, as does each child. What works for one child might not work for another. You might need to experiment a bit to find the best chair for your child. Here are some that parents have found that work for their children:

* A beanbag chair. Try an adult-size beanbag; some children love them.

* The Hang N' Seat from Right Start by U-Village straps onto a chair. It works well unless strapped to a chair that has a very high back. It is available at Target and other stores.

* The First Years On-the-Go Booster Seat works from ages 9 to 36 months and might work for a baby in a cast. It is available at Target and Babies "R" Us stores.

* Polly Highchair by Chicco. Some children in a spica cast can fit into this chair. It has soft padding on the sides.

* Ikea PS Brum children's armchair. This chair works for some children.

* Hammock chair. Some children love to sit in a hammock chair.

* Car seat. A portable car seat that is easily removed from its base might work as a chair for your child. Try a large car seat that is made for an older child and does not have sides. Use a pillow behind the child so that he can sit straight up. You might be able to put the car seat onto a regular chair so that the child can sit at the family table. Secure the car seat to the chair so that the child doesn't fall.

* Stool. For a child in a Petrie (Bachelor) cast, a stool works as a low chair.

One mother recommends this high chair for a child in a spica cast.

> I found a high chair that fits my daughter and her cast great—the Stokke Tripp Trapp [chair]. It is a bit pricey, but if you haven't bought a high chair yet, this will probably work for your spica baby and be a great high chair for them to use for many years. I would recommend trying it out in the store before you buy though. My daughter (seven months) now sits at the table with us. I don't have to strain my back to feed her anymore. **[HIP-BABY DISCUSSION GROUP]**

● Baby Bouncer

Ask your pediatric orthopedic doctor before using a bouncer. In some cases, babies being treated for hip dysplasia should not use them. A baby bouncer often attaches to the door frame. Make sure that you know what the weight limit is for the bouncer. A cast adds about five pounds. The E & I baby bungee bouncer has worked well for some babies (four months, up to 25 lbs.). It is available at the website www.babyuniverse.com.

● Spica Chair

A spica chair is a chair that is made to accommodate a child in a cast. Often, a flat play surface is included like a school desk with an area cut away for the cast. Figure 55 shows Josie Rose in a spica chair that is shaped like a teapot.

Josie Rose's mother made the chair pictured Figure 55 and has this to say about spica chairs:

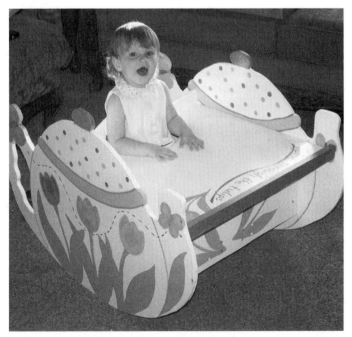

FIGURE 55. Josie Rose sitting in a spica chair *(Photo by Stephanie Micke)*

[Josie Rose] was the one who inspired me to create a special chair to allow her to sit up and reach her toys and feed herself. This chair made a tremendous difference in the way I was able to care for my daughter. She spent most of her day in her chair playing with her toys, coloring, watching her videos, and of course, rocking! It made the entire spica experience so much easier for both of us.

[STEPHANIE]

Stephanie created a business called IvyRose Spica chairs. If you are handy, you can build a chair. You can request instructions from the Our Tattered Angel blog or through the associated Facebook group. For more information about spica chairs and hip dysplasia blogs, see the Resources chapter on page 188.

● Making a Play Table

If you are handy, you can make adjustments to furniture that you already own or to inexpensive furniture that you buy. Use an inexpensive plastic table and chair set such as the Tender Heart Table and Chairs set from Little Tykes. Take the harness off the high chair and screw it onto one of the chairs. The child can sit in the chair and eat from the table. This table can be used with a chair or a stroller.

To make a play table:

1. Get an inexpensive wooden table for children.

2. Cut a semicircle where the child will sit.

3. Line the edges of the table with pool noodles so that toys will not fall off. Or try foam pipe insulation, which is available at hardware stores. For older children, the insulation must be attached.

● Making a Scooter Board for a Petrie (Bachelor) Cast

If you are handy you can build a scooter board to work with this cast (see Figure 56). The scooter board described in this section works better on hard surfaces than on carpet. It is made of thick foam on a board with wheels or casters. The child sits on the foam and the bar goes in the space between the pieces of foam. You can use a belt to strap the child in while riding.

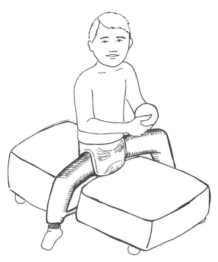

FIGURE 56. A child wearing a Petrie
(Bachelor) cast on a scooter board

Sleeping

The first night is the hardest, but it can take two to three weeks for a child to adjust to sleeping in a cast after surgery. Anesthesia could throw off his or her sleeping schedule for as long as three weeks. Here are some suggestions that might help ease the adjustment period:

Pain relief. Check with the doctor to confirm the best pain medicine and the dose for your child at bedtime. Some doctors recommend infant ibuprofen (Advil or Motrin) or acetaminophen (Tylenol) for pain, or Benadryl to make a child drowsy. Your child could be uncomfortable while his or her muscles stretch and adjust.

Prop up your child's legs and upper body. Use a rolled-up blanket or cushion under the child's legs, especially if one is dangling. As his or her muscles stretch, you can reduce the height of the props until he or she doesn't need them anymore. Also try a Memory Foam pillow. Some babies are comfortable tilted to the side with one or both legs propped up. It is helpful to elevate the head and upper body to help keep urine from leaking into the cast.

For a baby or young child, try a swing if the legs are supported. If the baby's legs are dangling, the cast might press against his or her skin. If you are not sure, check with your doctor.

Change your child's position. Your child might not be able to roll over. Given time, he or she might figure out how to roll over, even in a cast. You can turn your child over to make him or her more comfortable. Make sure that he or she can breathe easily, and take care with babies that no blankets are near the face.

Consider teething or other problems. If the child is inconsolable, the problem could be something else (not the hips). Check for the same things you would otherwise look for in a fussy child: teething for a baby or symptoms of a virus or an ear infection.

If you are worried about your child, check with your doctor. Some children don't sleep as well in the cast as they did before. One family put a recliner in their daughter's room because she did not sleep well while she was in the cast. If she was inconsolable, one of the parents would lie in the recliner with her until she calmed down.

Some health-care providers recommend moving a child in a spica cast even during the night. For a healthy child with hip dysplasia, this is not necessary. As Dr. Price from the IHDI medical board explains:

> The recommendation for frequent position changes is overemphasized for otherwise healthy children. We do see pressure sores in paralyzed patients or in debilitated patients who can't tell you when they are in an uncomfortable position. In those cases, the position should be shifted every two hours to allow blood circulation to the skin. Healthy children with hip dysplasia can wiggle enough in the cast to allow blood circulation or they will let you know when they are uncomfortable (mothers can tell). A comfortable position is my recommendation. A properly padded and positioned cast should protect the hip and allow comfort in almost any position. Simply tilting the cast every few hours is usually sufficient, and one position at night is usually fine if the child is resting comfortably. Pain at one spot can mean too much pressure there, so don't ignore pain, but it's pretty safe to ignore comfort.   **[CHARLES T. PRICE, MD]**

While Patti Sheeter's daughter Megan was in a cast, her family decided that she should sleep downstairs.

> Megan's bedroom was upstairs, so we moved her bed to our playroom/study downstairs. She was able to watch movies and play on the computer, and we didn't have to try to haul her up and down the stairs. The portable DVD player and Nintendo DS became our best friends! A small laptop, tablet, Kindle, etc. would have been great, too (but we didn't have those things). Megan also enjoyed playing Wii.   **[PATTI]**

Going Places

Keep as much of your routine from before the cast as you can. For example, if you usually go to story time at the library, then keep doing it. Bring your child to the grocery store with you. Make sure he or she still plays with friends. Some parents use infant slings (see "Slings and Baby Carriers" below) to carry a young child in a cast. If the child's cast makes it hard to sit, then a wagon with a few cushions could solve the problem.

● Slings and Baby Carriers

Check with your doctor before using a sling or baby carrier. He or she could have some guidelines about what positions your baby can be in while in treatment for hip dysplasia. Parents have had success carrying children in casts with the slings and baby carriers listed here. Other products might also work.

* Baby Bjorn carrier
* Ergo Baby carrier
* Kelty Kangaroo Infant Child Carrier, up to 28 lbs.
* Maya Wrap Baby Sling Baby Carrier, up to 35 lbs.
* Nojo Sling
* Playtex Deluxe Hip Hammock, 15–35 lbs.

● Strollers

Umbrella strollers often work well for a child in a cast. The legs can go over the side. With a stroller and some small pillows or rolled-up towels, you can take your child anywhere in a cast. You can even go grocery shopping. Push the stroller with one hand and pull the grocery cart behind you. It will do everyone some good to have a change of scenery and keep your child involved in family life. Some strollers and scooters that might work are listed here:

* Berchet Bubble Go Walker stroller
* McClaren Triumph or Techno stroller
* Step 2 Push Around Buggy
* The Playskool Step Start Walk 'n Ride
* Homemade scooter board for a child in a Bachelor cast (see "Making a Scooter Board for a Petrie (Bachelor) Cast" on page 142.)

● Ride-On Toys

A child wearing a cast can have fun with a ride-on toy and enjoy the opportunity to move without assistance. Figure 57 shows Claudia on a tricycle when she was wearing a spica cast.

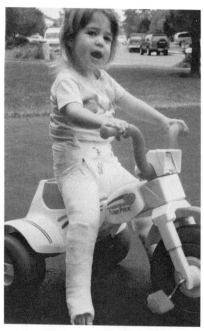

FIGURE 57. Claudia, age three, riding on a trike *(Photo courtesy of Nancy Sanders)*

Older children might use a wheelchair after surgery. Vivian describes how this worked with her daughter, Angela, who was diagnosed with hip dysplasia at the age of five:

Angela used a reclining wheelchair after both surgeries. It was the only option for her because she was cast in a reclining position. It was very large because her legs were spread pretty wide. I found it very easy to use and maneuver and believe it or not, not too heavy. I have a minivan so it easily fit in the back. I have four kids, one being a baby, so it was tricky not being able to use the stroller because we had to push the wheelchair. This year, my two girls fit in the wheelchair, and they ride together! **[VIVIAN]**

For more information about wheelchairs, see "Wheelchairs" on page 158.

How Other People React to Your Child

There will always be some people who stare when they see a child in a brace, harness, or cast. Bear in mind that they are probably trying to figure out what the baby or child is wearing and why. It is up to you whether you want to ignore this or offer a brief explanation. Older children might get embarrassed when people stare. A mother of a three-year-old has this to say about coping with comments:

Before the surgery, my daughter walked with a walker and braces. She was very self-conscious, but that was mostly because adults would stop in their tracks and stare and say things. Even though they were nice things like, "What a cute little girl," she didn't like it. Kids were easier, because they'd stop and ask what was wrong, and when they were told, they'd treat her normally.

I would practice a standard answer and teach it to her, such as "She had an operation and her leg is still healing." I would also talk to her preschool teachers. They can give you guidance about whether they think it is necessary to bring it up to the group. But honestly, my kid with all her accoutrements and inability to run around barely gets a second look. [HIP-BABY DISCUSSION GROUP]

Talk to your child about ways to respond when this happens. Children are often happy to be friends with a child in a cast, as Nancy's experience with neighborhood kids shows:

Make them a part of the solution and keep your daughter a part of the action. By that I mean tell the neighbor kids what is going on and ask them to help you. They can help by bringing balls over, letting your daughter throw them, and then they are the ones to retrieve the ball. Or else they can help by pushing her on a ride-on toy. One of our neighbor kids loved to push Claudia around on her fire truck (with me right behind, that is!).   [NANCY]

For information about older children attending school after treatment, see "Making Arrangements at School" on page 83.

School and Peers

Claudia had a severe case of hip dysplasia and had osteotomy surgery. Her mother, Nancy, a teacher herself, had this to say in response to a mother who was worried about her daughter starting preschool while still limping after hip surgery:

Many three-year-olds are not real keen on new people and situations. Take it slowly the first weeks when you drop her off. My daughter started preschool right after her osteotomies. She was unable to walk at that point, so the staff carried her everywhere. (Good thing she was a little peanut.) The other kids couldn't have cared less.

As the weeks went on and Claudia got stronger, she was able to walk a little bit, but still needed to be carried for long trips like to the playground and the lunchroom. The other kids took it in stride, and the teachers dealt with telling the curious when the need arrived. It was no big deal; it was just part of who Claudia was.

I would be up front with the teachers. A simple explanation such as, "She had surgery on her pelvis and femur, and she will limp because right now her legs are different lengths," should suffice. The preschool teachers should be able to help you and your daughter with the transition, without making your daughter feel bad.

[NANCY]

For children in elementary school, it might help for a parent to come into the classroom and explain what is going on. If you are able to do this, involve your child in planning and presenting this topic. This gives your child an opportunity to express himself or herself. Children often have strong preferences about certain things—even simple things like the color of a poster.

Checkups for a Child Wearing a Cast

A visit to the doctor's office while a child is in a cast usually does not take long. After taking an X ray to check the hips, the doctor sees if the child is outgrowing the cast. Discuss any questions you have during the doctor visit.

Wearing a cast might affect your child's vaccination schedule. Some shots are best given in the thigh instead of the arm. If it is important for a child to be vaccinated on schedule with a particular type of shot, the shot might be given in the child's buttocks, or the doctor can check with the manufacturer of the shots to make sure it is safe to give the shot in the arm instead. In some cases, the shots can be delayed until after the cast is removed.

When the Doctor Changes the Cast

Most children who wear a cast need to have one or more cast changes as they grow. In many cases, each new cast covers less of the child than the previous one. For example, the first cast could cover both legs completely. The second cast could stop above the knee on one or both legs. A cast change often takes less than an hour. A typical cast change goes like this:

1. Your child is given anesthesia so that he or she will stay still.
2. The old cast is removed.
3. The doctor applies a new cast.
4. An X ray might be taken to make sure that the hips are in the right position inside the cast.
5. Your child is moved to recovery.

When your child wakes up, he or she might not move his or her legs at first, even in a less-restrictive cast. The child will have dry skin and dead skin on the newly exposed parts of his or her legs. He or she might need pain relief such as acetaminophen (Tylenol) or ibuprofen (Advil or Motrin). Some children get muscle spasms in their legs, which might not occur until later when you are at home. If a child has muscle spasms, the doctor can prescribe medicine to treat them. See "Pain Management at Home" on page 97.

The shape of the hole in the cast could be larger or smaller than the previous cast. If your child wears diapers, try a diaper change at the doctor's office or hospital to make sure you are comfortable. The doctor tells you when to come back for the next cast checkup. After a second cast change, the child usually adjusts more quickly. He or she might test out how much more movement is possible or even try to stand.

When the Cast Comes Off

Tip: If you have a daughter, consider bringing loose long pants for her to wear on the car trip home. She will have dead skin on her legs that could get all over the car seat if she is wearing a dress.

If the child is wearing a plaster cast, the doctor uses a saw to cut apart the cast to remove it. The saw is loud and makes the cast vibrate, which tends to scare young children. Some hospitals have noise-dampening headphones that the child wears while the saw is being used. A fiberglass cast might be unwrapped instead of cut. That said, some children take it in stride, as shown in Figure 58.

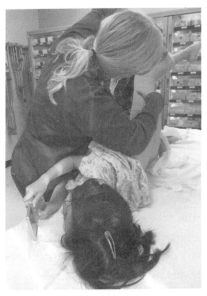

FIGURE 58. Megan playing with her
Gameboy while her cast is removed
(Photo courtesy of Patti Streeter)

Once the cast is off, the child's hips are X rayed. The doctor reviews the status of the hip with you—the structure and how he expects the hip to grow—what has improved since surgery, and what should come next. Many children wear a brace after the cast is removed. They see the doctor every four to six weeks and will do so as long as they are wearing the brace. These are some questions to ask the doctor when the cast comes off:

* Will my child be in a brace after the cast comes off?

* What type of brace?

* For how long will my child wear the brace?

* Will she wear the brace 24 hours a day, or will she be allowed out for some play time each day?

Adjusting to Life without a Cast

After the cast comes off, your child will have dry or scaly skin. Bathing helps, and some parents also like to use a cream. Some creams recommended by parents are Aquaphor products, or Healthy Times baby skin care products such as Honeysuckle baby bath and Sweet Violet lotion.

For the first week or more, your child could be in some pain and will be stiff. He might want to be held, and you might need to support his back while his muscles adjust and get stronger. Some children start kicking right away. For others it takes time for them to get used to the new freedom from the cast. Let your child be the one to decide when to move his legs. When you change his diaper, move slowly as he gradually loosens up. If the child wore a cast for a long time, his legs might stay in the same position, and only gradually will he be able to bring them closer together.

As a general rule, for each week of wearing a cast, allow a week of recuperation. So if a child was in a cast for eight weeks, it will most likely take eight weeks for him to get back to the level of strength that he had before the cast was put on. If your child is stiff and uncomfortable, warm baths can help. Put him in a bath chair so he can sit with support. This may help relax the muscles and improve flexibility. Note that some stiffness can actually be beneficial during healing because it can help keep the hip joint in a healthy alignment.

It can take months for a child to walk normally after major surgery such as an osteotomy. Your child might favor one side and might not want to be touched around the incision site. Try to be patient and let your child do as much on his own as possible. It is quicker to pick up and move a child but allow extra time when you can for the child to move at his own pace.

After this transition period, a young child will discover new ways to move such as rolling over or trying to crawl. If your child wears a brace after the cast, you might be surprised at what he can learn to do while wearing it. Some children learn to walk in it. With the increased activity, your child might eat more.

As your child begins to move, the hip joints could make snapping or popping sounds because they have been in the same position for so long. This is caused by tendons moving in the hip joint. It does not mean that the top of the thighbone is coming out of the hip socket. The sounds typically come and go, and it does not hurt your child when this happens. This is common, but if you are concerned, discuss it with your doctor.

Older children need to make adjustments when the cast comes off. The following quote describes a four-year-old girl who has been out of the spica for six weeks:

It is difficult in the beginning when they want to move but can't. We have a children's physiotherapist coming to the house who is really good with her. We offer daily rewards to her for completing the exercises. She also gave us a children's-size walker to use which my daughter rejected at first, but now uses because of the independence it gives her. When they've been in a spica for a long time, it takes a while for them to get adjusted to being without it. It almost becomes like a security blanket for them. Everyone thinks she would be so glad to get rid of it, but she's not! She still talks about having the cast on. It's so hard to know what's going through their minds, especially when they are older and just won't tell you how they are feeling. We've also been advised by the physio to start swimming.

[HIP-BABY DISCUSSION GROUP]

Wearing a Brace after a Cast

A brace is easier to manage than a cast. The child fits into car seats better. The type of brace used and the length of time it is worn depend on your child's individual treatment. The brace could be worn full-time, 18 hours a day, or only when your child sleeps. Compared to the cast, your child can move a lot more, but it will take some time for him or her to adjust. Be careful when you dress your child. Clothing with snaps on the legs might be easiest at first. Then you won't need to move the legs together to get pants on.

Some health insurance companies initially resist covering the cost of a brace worn after a spica cast is removed. If this happens, notify the insurance company that the brace is part of the total recovery plan; it is necessary to hold the hip in the right position over a period of time. A brace adds extra support when a cast is removed while a child is regaining muscle strength. If a brace is needed and the child does not wear it, then there is a greater chance that more surgery will be needed in the future. Sending a photograph of your child in the spica cast to the insurance company shows the extent of the procedure that your child underwent.

> After wearing a Pavlik harness for ten weeks, Sydney had a closed reduction, followed by a wearing spica cast for twelve weeks. Then she wore a Hewson brace at night and for naps. At Sidney's follow-up visit at the age of eight months, the news was very good.
>
> The pediatric orthopedic surgeon said her hips look "excellent." What a relief!
>
> Syd has been in a brace for nights and naps and will continue until she turns one. The surgeon said she is probably being overly cautious with the brace, which I welcome! Syd does not mind it either. Now it helps prepare her for sleep, and she crawls and rolls in it.
>
> She did so well in the spica and after. She rolled three days after she came out, and there has been no stopping her since. She sits up from her belly, crawls, and just last night pulled herself up on her legs while holding onto the couch. Our surgeon told us the cast would not delay her as long as we treated her like a normal baby when she came out, and, boy, was she right.   [JULIE]

Play and Physical Therapy

Most babies and young children do not need physical therapy after the cast is removed. Their everyday movements are enough for them to regain strength and mobility. If a child has missed milestones while in the cast, he or she gradually catches up. If a child in a spica cast was walking, he or she probably will not be able to walk at first when the cast is removed. If this happens, reassure the child that he or she will be able to walk again—it just takes time.

If your child does goes to physical therapy, the physical therapist evaluates how your child moves and selects exercises based on your child's individual situation. The physical therapist might work with certain muscle groups such as abdominal muscles or muscles in and around the hip joints. Some other areas that might come up are posture, gait, body awareness, position sensing, and muscle sense. Children with cerebral palsy (CP) and hip dysplasia might see an occupational therapist to work on sensory integration. Physical therapists who work with babies and young children use strategies like toy placement to encourage children to move.

● W-Sitting after Treatment

Some children like to sit with their legs in a W position (see Figure 59). This is called W-sitting.

Many children find this position comfortable and will move in and out of it while playing whether or not they have a history of hip dysplasia treatment. In the past, many medical professionals thought this position could cause unstable hips. Now, it is believed to be a result of the child's hip structure, rather than a cause.

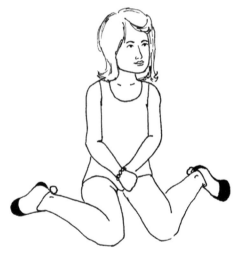

FIGURE 59. A child, W-sitting

If your child has low muscle tone and sits this way often, it can stress the knees and hips. He or she might need to learn to sit other ways. Talk to your doctor to find out if your child needs help from a physical therapist. Also see "Low Muscle Tone" on page 38.

Regaining Muscle Strength

Most young children do not need physical therapy after wearing a cast. Normal movement is usually enough for a child to regain strength and range of motion. For those children who need some extra help, the physical therapist usually encourages the child to try normal everyday movements. For example, a baby might be placed on his or her stomach, even if is only for 30-second intervals at first. This encourages the baby to roll over. Or a toy might be placed just out of reach so that the child has to stretch to get it.

After the cast is removed, most children gradually start to move their legs down and closer together. This allows them to crawl and to stand. Even if your child walked while wearing a cast, he or she probably will not be able to walk at first when the cast comes off. If your child has a very wide stance for more than a month, check with your pediatric orthopedic doctor or physical therapist (if your child has one). Though parents sometimes worry that about a stiff hip, this initial stiffness can actually hold the hip in a good position that is beneficial to the hip-joint development.

9
Recovery for Older Children and Adolescents

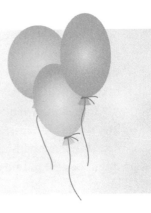

Older children and teens do not wear a cast after surgery for hip dysplasia. Typically they use a wheelchair and walking aids, such as crutches or a walker, while they are recovering. Before your child or teen goes home, the hospital staff will teach him or her how to safely use the walker or crutches.

Preparing Your Home

Before your child comes home, remove throw rugs and clutter to minimize tripping hazards. It's a good idea to stock up on groceries and to cook some meals ahead of time and freeze them.

Plan for your child to sleep downstairs if you have stairs in your home. Some people like to use a hospital bed for the first few weeks. A hospital bed makes it easier to change position, and the trapeze bar makes it easier to get in and out of bed. Some homes, however, do not have enough room for a hospital bed.

A raised toilet seat makes it much easier for an older child or young adult to use the bathroom at home. Some hospitals provide them. The doctor might write a prescription for it at a medical supply store, which might be covered by your health insurance. Ask about this before surgery in case you need to arrange to get the toilet seat yourself. The most versatile kind of raised toilet seat can be used both by the bedside and over the toilet. Find out if the hospital will provide this, or if you need to order it. Baby wipes might work better than toilet paper when your child first comes home. Have some on hand just in case.

Your child will be allowed to take showers before he or she is allowed to take a bath. A shower bench or chair and a handheld showerhead can make bathing easier. If you have a walk-in shower, then you might be able to find a raised toilet seat that also works as a shower chair.

The physical therapist or occupational therapist at the hospital can recommend other equipment and tools to aid you and your child during recovery. Tools such as a grabber to pick up things, put on socks, etc., make everyday tasks a little easier.

Helping Your Child with Movement

The physical therapist at the hospital will help your child learn safe ways to move while protecting the hip that had surgery. The hospital staff should also go over this with you. After you get home, there may be some instances when your child needs help, especially the first time he or she tries to do something.

Here are a few ideas to keep in mind with these firsts. Ask your child if he or she wants help or would rather try to move while you stand by just in case. If your child wants you to help move the leg on the operated side, make sure he or she is ready and then move slowly, following any movement restrictions that the doctor has given you. Moving the leg suddenly can be painful to your child.

Wheelchairs

Wheelchairs come in pediatric or adult sizes, and some can recline, which is useful if the doctor recommends a semireclining position during recovery. Your child might be able to use a wheelchair to eat with the family at the dining room table. Most wheelchairs can be collapsed when not in use.

Ask the hospital staff to show you how to push your child in the wheelchair. The staff also can show you how to set the brakes and

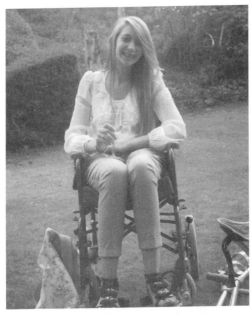

FIGURE 60. Emily using a wheelchair after femoral osteotomy surgery *(Photo courtesy of Emily Marrows)*

how to fold and open the wheelchair. Pushing a wheelchair is similar to pushing a stroller. Older children can move their own wheelchairs, but there may be times when they need help, especially if they are very tired due to surgery and the effects of pain medications.

When going up a ramp, push the wheelchair as you normally would. To go down a ramp, turn around so that both you and your child have your backs to the bottom of the ramp. Then carefully walk backward down the ramp as you pull the wheelchair after you.

To go up a curb, line up the front of the wheelchair so that both front wheels touch the curb at the same time. Tilt the wheelchair back a bit so the front wheels can go up the curb. Then bring the chair to a level position as you push the back wheels up onto the curb. To go down a curb, turn the wheelchair so that both you and your child have your back to the curb. Step down, and then carefully pull the wheelchair after you so that the rear wheels go down the curb first.

To load a wheelchair into the trunk of a car:

1. If the wheelchair is too heavy for you, ask for help.

2. Remove any small parts that can come off such as cushions.

3. Fold the wheelchair (usually you pull the seat up to do this).

4. Using both hands, lift the wheelchair.

5. Slide the rear wheels in first.

6. Load any small parts that you have removed from the wheelchair.

Personalizing a Wheelchair, Crutches, or a Walker

After hip surgery, your child uses a wheelchair and a walking aid such as crutches or a walker until he or she is cleared by the doctor to walk independently. Some people like to decorate these items. Decorations can be as simple as applying colorful duct tape or stickers to crutches, or they can be elaborate as shown in Figure 61.

There are companies like crutcheze.com and krutchpack.com that make items designed to work with crutches. Another company

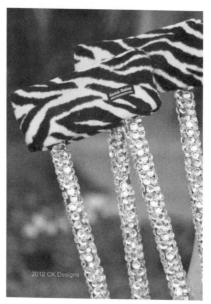

FIGURE 61. Cynthia decorated her daughter Bri's crutches. *(Photo courtesy of Cynthia Keenan)*

called Shrinkins sells decorative "skins" that can be temporarily applied to a walking aid and, later, easily removed. If you like the idea of decorating, but you are renting a wheelchair, you and your child could decorate it with a range of patterns from butterflies to skulls. Then you could remove the decorations before you return the equipment.

Incision Care

The doctor uses one of several methods to close the incision made during surgery: clips (like staples), stitches, or medical glue like Dermabond. The incision might have a bandage or dressing on it. Follow the doctor's instructions about caring for the incision site. This is sometimes called wound care. Though children are routinely given antibiotics during and after surgery to prevent infection, you are given instructions about how to spot an infection if it does occur—such as pain, redness, pus, or a temperature. If you think your child has an infection, call the doctor so that it can be treated.

If clips or stitches were used to close the incision, they are removed about ten days after surgery unless dissolving stitches were used. They don't have to be removed. You might be told to keep your child's incision dry for a certain period of time.

As the incision heals, a scar develops. The appearance of the scar can continue to change for up to a year after the surgery.

Nutrition and Healing

Children tend to heal well from surgery, though they might not feel like eating much for the first week or so afterward. You might have been told to stop all medicines and supplements for a couple of weeks before your child's surgery. It is important to follow the doctor's guidelines about that, but after surgery, when your child starts eating again, a multivitamin won't hurt and might be beneficial. The American Academy of Pediatrics recommendation is that all children need 400 IU of vitamin D supplementation. Vitamin D is beneficial to bones, and Vitamin C improves bone healing. Vitamin K is important for coagulation. Vitamin E increases bleeding time and should probably be avoided.

Periacetabular Osteotomy (PAO) Recovery and Physical Therapy

This section describes a typical recovery path after PAO surgery, which can be used to treat adolescents with hip dysplasia. If your child has a different kind of osteotomy, the recovery process is different. For a PAO or any other osteotomy surgery, the doctor develops a plan for each individual child. The doctor takes into consideration the specific surgery that is done and the child's age and adjusts the plan as needed as your child heals.

After PAO surgery, a physical therapist teaches your teen how to safely move and how to do simple exercises while protecting the affected hip as it heals. It is important to follow instructions for movement and physical therapy exercises to minimize pain and inflammation during the healing process. Though each teen has his or her own physical therapy program, from a big-picture point of view, the recovery path after a PAO can be divided into four phases. Bear in mind that the length of each phase is an estimate. Depending on their individual plan, some people will spend a longer or shorter amount of time in each phase than the examples included here.

● *Phase 1: Weeks 1–6*

This phase starts in the hospital the first day after surgery (see "Postoperative (Post-Op) Recovery at the Hospital" on page 93). Physical therapy begins with exercises that can be done while lying down, such as ankle pumps (point and flex the feet), and exercises that use the quadriceps muscles in the front of the thigh.

Your teen uses crutches or a walker and does not bear weight on the operated side. The foot on the operated side touches down lightly. When walking, a step-to gait is used in which the foot on the side that had surgery moves forward first with the walker or crutches. Then, while the arms support the body, the other foot is brought up next to the first foot. The exception to this method is when ascending stairs, in which case the leg on the side without surgery goes up first. Some people use the phrase, "up with the good" to remember this.

After your teen comes home, he or she continues to work with a physical therapist either at home or at a physical therapy facility. Posture and alignment during exercises are more important than the number of repetitions that can be done. In addition to muscles that were directly affected by the surgery, it is possible that, before surgery, your teen's muscles were compensating for a shallow hip socket. If this was the case, some muscles might be stronger than usual, and others might be weaker than usual. It takes time and practice to learn new, more balanced ways of using these muscles.

● Phase 2: Weeks 6–12

During this phase, your teen gradually begins to bear weight on the leg on the side that had hip surgery. He or she learns to go up and down a step and to balance on one foot. Posture and gait continue to be important. The goal is to use a healthy gait with good posture so that by the end of this phase, crutches or a walker are not needed. This phase has no universal set of exercises because the doctor and physical therapist select exercises appropriate for each individual. Some physical therapy exercises that might be recommended are: leg presses, squats, and heel slides. Your teen might use elastic bands for some exercises.

● Phase 3: Weeks 12–16

The physical therapist continues to work with your teen to increase the range of motion in the hip joint without going beyond healthy positions (overextending the joint). Exercises are used to build strength while maintaining good balance. Your teen might be allowed to go to the gym, to use an elliptical machine, and to ride a bike.

● Phase 4: Weeks 16–20

During this phase your teen moves toward an independent exercise program while minimizing soreness. By the end of this phase, your teen might be allowed to run and engage in many physical activities or sports. The goal is to engage in these activities without pain, so your teen will be given guidance about how to become increasingly active and to minimize the risk of injuries at the same time.

Total Hip Replacement (THR) Recovery

It is very rare for teenagers to undergo total hip replacement (THR) surgery (see "Total Hip Replacement (THR)" on page 115). A teen would need to have finished growing. The surgery and recovery process for a teen who has a THR is similar to what a young adult goes through. This section gives an overview of what THR recovery entails. For more detailed information, please see the book *A Guide for Adults with Hip Dysplasia* (West and Sutherland).

Whether the implant that goes into the femur is cemented or cementless affects how soon the teen or young adult can bear weight after the surgery. With a cemented implant, it is possible to bear weight within two or three days. If a cementless implant was put in, the teen or young adult might be instructed to use partial weight bearing or toe-touch weight bearing for six weeks.

The doctor specifies movement restrictions, such as not crossing the legs and not bending more than 90 degrees when sitting, which vary according to the individual's surgery and typically last about three months. The movement restrictions prevent the artificial hip from dislocating as the body heals. The teen or young adult will have a physical therapy program. This begins in the hospital with simple exercises that can be done lying down and gradually increases in difficulty as the teen or young adult heals and regains his or her strength.

Getting Through Recovery

The recovery process after surgery for hip dysplasia takes an extended period of time. This can be frustrating, but it is impressive how people do manage to adapt and find the strength and stamina required. The following sections provide different points of view about recovery.

● *Teen Voices*

In this section, some teens have generously offered to share their thoughts about their experiences with surgery for hip dysplasia.

Emily, who had femoral osteotomies, has this to say about her experience.

In my experience of the whole journey, I have really had a roller coaster of experiences and emotions. People treated me very differently because I looked a normal teenage girl but in a wheelchair, often asked if it was for a joyride or because I couldn't be bothered to walk, but people didn't realize how upset and sensitive I was.

The journey didn't start the day of my operation; it started the day I was diagnosed, and I will have a constant reminder through life due to my scarring and the pain. It is so frustrating for both me and my mum that we have been ignored for 15 years [Emily was misdiagnosed with growing pains], when this could have all been avoided.

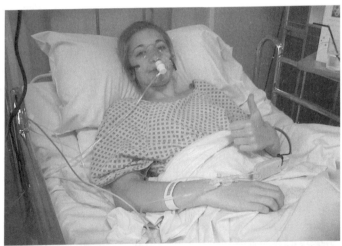

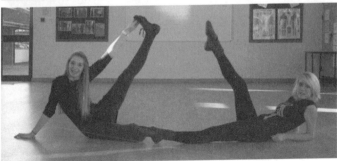

FIGURE 62. Emily before surgery and after recovery *(Photos courtesy of Emily Marrows)*

I found it all very difficult to handle at first because shop assistants would often talk down to me, as if they were more superior to me. Words cannot describe how hard it was for me and my family. Being a dancer, it was hard to get back into things, especially knowing how far I could push myself and get back to dancing. But hopefully the future will get brighter, and I will get back to being the old me.

I'd advise other teens who need surgery to listen to the consultants[4]—and doctors—if they say to rest then rest and not try as get back to normal and overdo anything, not to suffer. Take the pain relief. Also, don't listen to the scary things that people tell you because everyone is different, and it's not as bad as everyone makes out.

[EMILY]

Bri had PAO surgery, later had her pins removed, and then had another surgery to remove some excess bone that had grown in her hip. Here is what she has to say:

I had built my whole life around cheerleading. Before my surgery I tried to talk to my friends, but they didn't know what to say. No one understood. I'd tell them about the surgery, and they'd say they were sorry and then the conversation would end. My best friend from fourth grade stopped being my friend. I was shocked. Maybe we would have branched off anyway, but it was really hard. I was so angry. People would post in their [Facebook] status that they had the worst day, and I would feel like they had no right to complain.

The first week after surgery was hard. School was in session, so I couldn't phone people to talk to them. When I went back to school, I attended part-time. The other students didn't understand the severity of the situation. They would see me in some classes and not others, so they assumed I was fine. Some people would ask, "Why aren't you at school?" in a rude tone, implying that I was lazy. That was upsetting.

Without cheerleading practice, I had no friends to hang out with. They were forgetting about me. I did reach out to other people, but we didn't have as much in common. My family was helpful and supportive. I had to adapt. I'm more cautious now, and I sometimes separate myself from friends. I've grown as a person. I turned to school since I could still do academic subjects. I want to study neuroscience.

I'd really advise other teens to stay positive. It might seem like there are a million reasons to frown, but there's always gonna be at least one reason to smile, and they should really focus on that. It's a lot harder emotionally than most people would expect. I wish I was a little more prepared in that aspect. I did however focus on academics a lot to distract my mind, which was incredibly helpful. [BRI]

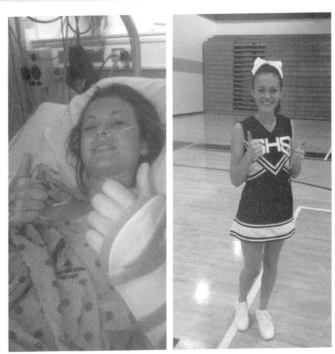

FIGURE 63. Bri before and after her surgeries *(Photos courtesy of Bri Keenan)*

Happy Hips is a group of teens with hip dysplasia. They offer the following suggestions for parents and teens when dealing with surgery for hip dysplasia.

Happy Hips Tips for Parents:

* Let your child know you are always there for him or her.

* Try and find a group to join online or a contact through charities to learn from other parents' experiences.

* Suggest to your child someone he or she can speak to such as—one of your friends whom he or she knows well, a family member, or a counselor—who is impartial and will not tell you about the conversation. Sometimes teens feel unable to talk to their parents about certain aspects of this journey and simply need someone else to turn to.

* It's sometimes necessary to be firm to keep your child on track.

* Plan little treats for your child out of the blue just because you know it will cheer him or her up.

Happy Hips Tips for Teenage Hippies:

* Talk to others and express your concerns.

* Try to contact another teen who has been through this experience or even someone who's at a similar stage in the process.

* Keep thinking positively.

* Remember sometimes you just have to accept that you can't do something yet and, instead, look forward to the time when you will be able to do it. Also adapt and find new activities that you could try, such as reading new books and a bit of craft instead of playing impact sports, etc.

* Remember that you are not alone!!

[THE HAPPY HIPS TEAM]

● *Thoughts from a Physical Therapist*

Kelly Ariagno is a physical therapist who had PAO surgery as an adult and has worked with patients recovering from PAO surgery. She offers the following advice about the ups and downs involved in recovery:

It's perfectly normal to have a string of good days or bad days when you feel stronger, mobile, or pain-free versus feeling sore, weak, tired, or stiff. Your body needs plenty of time to heal, adapt to new activities, and adjust to the new alignment of your hip. Remember, your hip socket has been realigned and your muscles are adapting to new lengths and positions. It may take a full year before you feel very comfortable with your "new hip."

It's helpful to expect ups and downs and various changes in sensation over time so that you don't feel frustrated or scared when you seem to be taking a step backward. However, if you experience any significant changes in your condition that worry you or if you are not improving, certainly contact your surgeon or physical therapist.

[KELLY]

● Emotional and Mental Health

The previous section described some of the physical ups and down that occur during the recovery process. The recovery process also has emotional and mental challenges to get through. Encourage your child to talk to you about how she is doing. If she reports being in pain or feeling that something is wrong, believe her. Some children want to please parents and be the "perfect patient." In this case, the child might hesitate to speak up if something is wrong to avoid disappointing you. This can happen with children who are "people pleasers." These children tend also to be perfectionists and are more prone to anxiety.

Adolescence is a time of developing a sense of self and identity. If your child is athletic, he or she will have to reinvent his or her identity as an athlete in the context of sports and physical activity after surgery. This also affects the social side of things if your child's friends are centered around a particular sport or physical activity.

This surgery has a long recovery period. Even if your child is able to return to school weeks after surgery, it could take a couple of months before he is able to fully absorb lessons and to be as socially active as before. Peer groups fluctuate a lot in middle school and high school, even without the hip surgery issue. It's common to lose some friends and make new ones. Losing friends can be especially painful if that coincides with surgery, and it might make the child hesitant about trying to make new friends. If this happens, it might be easier to connect with others in structured social settings such as clubs. If your child experiences bullying at school or cyberbullying, seek out support for your child. Cyberbullying can continue to affect kids even when they are not physically in school (when they are out due to surgery).

Dr. Fan, a child, adolescent, and adult psychiatrist and pediatrician has the following to say about the psychological issues in connection with hip surgery and recovery for older children and teens:

Worries, fears, and anxiety about the surgery, pain, recovery period, and the outcomes are to be expected. When there is not a proper outlet for these feelings, it's possible that they may be expressed outwardly as irritability, anger, or panic attacks, or they can manifest as depressed mood or somatic pain [pain without a medical cause].

Erikson's work describes the adolescent stage (ages thirteen to nineteen) as identify vs. role confusion.[5] The additional stressors of the diagnosis, surgery, and disability (even if temporary) are significant during this stage. Here is what you can do to help your teens:

1. Going to the basics: proper nutrition and adequate sleep and rest are the key to mental health.

2. Be supportive and be there for your child. Support (emotionally and educationally advocating for your child) is essential to help during this time of transition.

3. Help your teen maintain a connection to other teens. Having supportive peer groups is one of the protective factors during adolescence. In addition to friends, teens may find clubs and support groups (meeting other teens with hip dysplasia) to be helpful.

4. Encourage your teen to explore hobbies or interests that are not physically demanding, such as writing or journaling, arts and crafts, music, and reading. These activities can be very helpful during this period. Maybe you could do something fun to-

➡

gether as a family such as watching a movie or having a family
game night.

5. Make professional help available to your child. Participating in
counseling sessions can provide a safe place for teens to talk
about their concerns and feelings and work through conflicts.
Sometimes family sessions can help with communication and
strengthen relationships.

6. Take care of yourself. Sometimes parents forget that their own
health (both physical and mental) is the foundation to the family and their children's well-being. Parents support groups can
be very helpful as well.

The following signs and symptoms are associated with depression and anxiety in children:

* Depression: Low mood, irritability, loss of interests, crying for
no reason, sleep changes (more or less), appetite changes
(more or less), weight gain or loss, feeling worthless or guilt,
low energy, poor concentration, helplessness, hopelessness,
and thoughts about death or suicide.

* Anxiety: Irritability, worries, fears, muscle tension, panic symptoms.

* Somatic symptoms (aches and pains without medical causes)
are also quite frequent with anxiety and depression.

If you have any concerns about your child's physical and mental well-being, it's important to seek professional help immediately.

[KATHERINE FAN, MD]

Many of the physical symptoms associated with depression (sleep
changes, appetite changes, low energy, low concentration) are normal within the context of post-op recovery. Some children are ane-
mic after surgery, so they are very tired. Note that muscle tension is
different from the muscle spasms that can also occur after hip surgery. For physical symptoms, your child's doctor can explain what to
expect as your child heals.

A certain amount of anxiety and sadness is to be expected during
recovery, both in the child who is healing from surgery and in

parents who are caring for the child. There is nothing wrong with crying when there is a reason to cry. Problems occur if sadness settles in and never seems to lift, if feelings go beyond ordinary sadness, or if anxiety escalates as described in Dr. Fan's quote. If you are worried about your child's mood, contact your child's doctor to discuss the situation.

● Parent Perspectives

Amanda's daughter, Emily, was diagnosed with hip dysplasia as a teen. You can read Emily's advice to other teens in the "Teen Voices" section above. Amanda and Emily had the very frustrating experience of bringing up Emily's leg pain to doctors for years, only to be told the problem was growing pains. After Emily was referred to a consultant (a specialist in the United Kingdom), she had a femoral osteotomy (FVO) for each hip with the surgeries spaced apart. Amanda has this to say about some of the hardest parts for her as a parent.

> I work at our local hospital and see patients' scars every day, but it never prepared me for seeing Emily with eight-inch scars. Emily has keloid scarring which is very thick and raised. Emily doesn't like touching her scars, so when I rub bio oil on her, I feel upset because it could have been avoided if our doctor had listened to me.
>
> I found taking Emily shopping in her wheelchair hard. Shop assistants really treated her different because of her wheelchair. Emily is a pretty girl and obviously looks normal. They ignored her when she went to buy anything, so I would push her wheelchair to the counter and turn my back to the assistants so they had to talk to Emily.   [AMANDA]

Cynthia's daughter, Bri, was diagnosed with hip dysplasia as a teen. You can read Bri's comments in the "Teen Voices" section, too. Cynthia has this to say about her experience as a parent with the treatment Bri went through for developmental dysplasia of the hip (DDH):

It has been eighteen months since my daughter was diagnosed with DDH. Since then she has undergone a labral tear repair, PAO surgery on her right hip, hardware removal [of pins from the PAO], and arthroscopic surgery to remove heterotopic [excess] bone. There have been many ups and downs along the way, and I believe each person's journey is very unique.

The emotional part of the journey is tricky. I'm a "fixer," as I believe most moms are, and seeing your child in physical and emotional pain is extremely difficult. It continues to humble me.

What I can tell you at this point is that for all the stress and psychological highs and lows that come with a diagnosis of DDH, your child will emerge as pretty much the same person she was before. Bri has always been a happy and funny girl. But the months before the bone growth removal were pretty dark. She had already gone through so much and now this? It just didn't seem fair. Not to me, and certainly not to her. She was angry and frustrated and did not want to talk while I struggled with finding words to ease her mind.

In the midst of it, I received some great advice from our surgeon's nurse. She told me to just let her be. This was a setback, and she shouldn't be expected to be happy. It was only going to take time. So, Bri watched a lot of TV. We rented full seasons of the shows she likes, and she watched them nonstop, sometimes with us, sometimes alone, and sometimes for hours on end. She did extensive research on colleges and her intended major and planned a trip to visit several of them after her surgery. She became much more introverted and spent a lot of time alone. She did not want to see friends. I stopped encouraging her to invite people over and even let her miss a few family celebrations. She wasn't up to socializing at all, and I tried to protect her from it.

There were times I had my doubts that this was a healthy approach. I only share that because I'm so happy to report that my doubts were unfounded. Almost right out of her latest surgery, she's been laughing, joking, and enjoying life so much more. We visited the top five colleges on her list while she was still on crutches and a hip brace. She's making plans for her future and seems just as happy and funny as she's always been. Her DDH has been a difficult part of her life, but she's determined to not let it define her.   [CYNTHIA]

Notes

1. R. Wynne-Davis, "Acetabular Dysplasia and Familial Joint Laxity: Two Etiological Factors in Congenital Dislocation of the Hip," *Journal of Bone and Joint Surgery, British* 52-B, no. 4 (1970 November): 704–16.
2. M. J. Frantzen et al., "Gonad Shielding in Paediatric Pelvic Radiography: Disadvantages Prevail Over Benefit," *Insights Imaging* 3, no. 1 (February 2012): 23–32.
3. G. H. Prosser et al., "Outcome of Primary Resurfacing Hip Replacement: Evaluation of Risk Factors for Early Revision," *Acta Orthopaedica* 81, no. 1 (February 2010): 66–71.
4. In the United Kingdom, doctors who are specialists are called consultants.
5. Erik Erikson was a psychologist who described eight stages of development that people pass through during the course of a lifetime.

Glossary

abductor muscles. The muscles that move the legs outward.

acetabular dysplasia. The hip socket is not the right shape, and stays that way, which makes the hip unstable.

acetabular index (AI). The angle of hip socket between the bottom of the pelvis and the outer edge of the hip socket.

acetabulum. The hip socket, or the area in the pelvis that is capable of becoming a hip socket in a baby. Newborns have cartilage in this area. As the baby grows, this area becomes bone (ossifies).

adductor muscles. The muscles located across the groin that move the legs together (inward).

adductor tenotomy. Surgery in which the doctor nicks or cuts the adductor tendon so that the top of the thighbone can go into the hip socket. This is often done during a reduction.

ALARA. An abbreviation for "as low as is reasonably achievable." When X rays are taken, health-care workers use this guideline to minimize the amount of radiation used.

anesthesiologist. A doctor who completed an internship and residency in anesthesiology and is certified by the American Board of Anesthesiologists.

anterior approach. Surgery in which the doctor approaches the joint from the front.

anteversion. See *femoral anteversion.*

arthrogram. (arthography) An X ray with dye injected into a joint.

arthrogryposis. A rare congenital disorder that causes multiple joint contractures.

arthroscope. A surgical tool with a probe and a light. It lets the doctor make a small cut and view the structure of the hip joint.

arthroscopy. A surgical procedure sometimes used to repair tears in the labrum (the rim of soft tissue around the hip socket) for adults with hip dysplasia.

avascular necrosis of the hip (AVN). Also called osteonecrosis, aseptic necrosis, or ischemic bone necrosis. A loss of blood flow to the hip that results in bone death of the bone in the ball at the top of the femur.

Bachelor cast. A cast with a bar between the legs, also called a Petrie cast or a broomstick cast.

ball-and-socket joint. A joint that has a ball shape that fits inside a cup shape, such as the shoulder or hip.

Barlow's test. A hip exam used for babies to see if the hip is dislocatable.

bilateral. Affecting both sides.

bursitis. Irritation in the bursa, a fluid-filled sac that acts as a cushion between joint surfaces.

center edge (CE) angle. Used to diagnose the hip structure of children under eight years of age. It is the angle between the lateral border of the hip socket and a vertical line through the center of the femoral head. Normal is an angle greater than 25 degrees.

central core disease. A rare neurological disorder, usually inherited, in which the muscle cells contain cores.

closed reduction. A surgery in which the doctor moves the top of the thighbone into the hip socket without making an incision (cut).

clubfoot. A disorder in which the foot is turned downward and inward at birth and remains in this position.

collagen. A strong, fibrous protein in connective tissues and bones.

computed tomography (CT). A type of X ray in which the X-ray beam moves around the body so that images can be seen from many angles.

congenital. Present at birth.

congenital dysplasia of the hip (CDH). Hip dysplasia that is present at birth.

contralateral hip. The opposite hip.

coxalgic gait. Walking with a limp because of hip pain.

coxa magna. Condition in which the ball at the top of the thighbone (femoral head) is enlarged.

computer tomography (CT). A three-dimensional X ray that shows "slices."

developmental dysplasia of the hip (DDH). A condition in which the ball at the top of the thighbone (femoral head) is not in the correct position in the hip socket (acetabulum).

dislocatable hip. The top of the thighbone can move out of the hip socket.

dislocated (luxated) hip. The top of the thighbone is outside the hip socket.

Down syndrome. A chromosomal disorder in which all or part of an extra 21st chromosome is present.

epidural. Pain medicine that is given through a soft tube, called a catheter, into the epidural space, which is near the backbone and spinal cord.

femur. The thighbone.

femoral anteversion. The thighbone (femur) is twisted inward, causing the knees and toes to point inward.

femoral head. The ball at the top of the femur (thighbone).

femoral osteotomy. Surgery involving cutting the femur (thighbone), usually combined with repositioning it within the hip socket.

frank breech position. Inside the uterus, the baby's buttocks are positioned by the birth canal, and the baby's legs are straight up so that his or her feet are near the head.

Galeazzi test. A hip exam used for babies and young children to check for a dislocated hip on one side.

gastric reflux (GER). Spitting up. The stomach contents come back up through the esophagus. This is common in babies.

gastroesophageal reflux disease (GERD). A more serious form of gastric reflux.

geneticist. A doctor who has studied genetics and is certified by the American Board of Medical Genetics.

glucosamine chondroitin. A supplement that is sometimes recommended to help maintain cartilage in adults who have joints in which the cartilage is wearing out.

Graf scale. One method that doctors use to interpret infant hip ultrasounds.

hip abduction orthosis. A brace that is used to keep a child's hips in an abducted position (out to the sides).

hip resurfacing. This is a surgical alternative to total hip replacement (THR) surgery for some adults with hip problems. The femoral head and the hip socket are resurfaced, and metal implants are inserted.

hydrocolloidal bandage. A special kind of bandage made for open sores or burns.

hypermobility. Joints that can stretch farther than normal.

ischemic bone necrosis. See *avascular necrosis of the hip.*

incentive spirometer. A device used to encourage a patient to breathe deeply after surgery.

incision. The cut a doctor makes in order to do surgery.

irreducible. The top of the thighbone is outside the hip socket and cannot be reduced (it cannot go back inside the hip socket).

labrum. The rim of soft tissue that surrounds the hip joint.

leg-length discrepancy. One leg is longer than the other.

ligaments. Bands of tough tissue that connect bones together.

low muscle tone. Poor muscle tone, less strength than usual.

MRI (magnetic resonance imaging). MRI uses a strong magnetic field and radio waves to create images of tissues.

medial approach. Surgery in which the doctor approaches the joint from the side.

medial circumflex femoral artery (MFA). The artery that provides blood flow to the hip.

nonsteroidal anti-inflammatory drug (NSAID). These drugs offer pain relief and reduce inflammation. Some common examples are ibuprofen and aspirin.

open reduction. Surgery in which the doctor must make an incision (cut) in order to put the ball at the top of the thighbone inside the hip socket.

orthopedist. A doctor who treats problems with muscles and bones. Also see *pediatric orthopedic surgeon.*

orthotist. An orthotist makes and fits orthopedic harnesses and braces prescribed by doctors.

Ortolani test. A hip exam used for newborns to see if the hip is dislocatable.

ossification. The process of cartilage hardening into bone. This is a normal development in babies.

osteonecrosis. See *avascular necrosis of the hip.*

osteotomy. Surgery that involves cutting bone. Also see *pelvic osteotomy,* and *femoral osteotomy.*

osteoarthritis. A joint disease in which the cartilage wears away or breaks down, causing pain and inflammation.

patient-controlled anesthesia (PCA). Pain medication in a pump that is controlled by a patient, who pushes a button as needed to get more pain medicine.

Pavlik harness. A soft brace used for babies up to six months of age who have hip dysplasia.

pediatric orthopedic surgeon. A doctor who treats problems with muscles and bones in babies and children.

pediatrician. A doctor who specializes in treating children.

pelvic osteotomy. Cutting and reshaping the pelvis (bone) so that it holds the femoral head in the hip socket.

percent coverage. The amount of coverage that the hip socket provides for the femoral head (the ball at the top of the thighbone).

periacetabular osteotomy. A type of pelvic osteotomy surgery sometimes used for adolescents or adults with hip dysplasia to improve the structure of the hip joint.

petalling. A method of applying tape around the opening of a cast.

Petrie cast. Also called a Bachelor cast or broomstick cast. A cast with a bar between the legs.

physical therapist. A physical therapist is trained to work with people of all ages to prevent the onset, or reduce the progression, of conditions resulting from disease, injury, or other causes.

positional plagiocelphaly. A common condition experienced by babies in which part of the head becomes flat because the baby lies in the same position for too long.

posterior approach. Surgery in which the doctor approaches the joint from the back.

prostaglandins. Hormones that produce inflammation and pain.

pulvinar. Unwanted tissue within the hip joint, which may be fatty or fibrous. During an open reduction, this may need to be removed so that the femoral head can go into the hip socket.

radiologist. A medical doctor who is certified as a specialist in reading X rays, MRIs, and CT scans.

reduction. Putting a bone back into its proper position. Also see *closed reduction* and *open reduction*.

relaxin. A hormone that pregnant women produce, which relaxes their ligaments. Babies who are sensitive to this hormone can be born with lax ligaments.

remodeling. An ongoing normal process in which new bone gradually grows and old bone tissue is absorbed.

risk factors. Reasons why a person is more likely to have a medical condition.

scoliosis. A condition in which the spine is curved.

shelf procedure. A type of osteotomy surgery in which bone is added at the top of the hip socket to add support to the joint.

spica cast. A body cast that is used to hold a child's hips in place after a closed or open reduction.

spina bifida. A birth defect affecting the spinal cord that involves the neural tube.

subluxated hips. A condition in which there is some contact between the femoral head and the hip socket.

synovial fluid. The fluid within a joint that lubricates it.

synovial lining. Also called synovium, the lining of a joint such as the hip joint.

talipes equinovarus. See *clubfoot*.

tenotomy. Surgery in which the doctor makes a small cut to allow a tendon to stretch farther. This is sometimes done together with a reduction.

tendons. The connective tissues that attach muscles to bones.

teratologic dislocations. One or both hips did not develop properly before the baby was born. The hips are dislocated and the top of the thighbone cannot be moved into the hip socket.

toeing in. See *femoral anteversion.*

toeing out. The feet turn outward toward the sides.

total hip replacement (THR). Surgery in which the top of the thighbone (femoral head) and the corresponding part of the hip socket are replaced with an implant.

traction. Weights and pulleys used to stretch muscles.

transducer. A handheld device used during ultrasound.

Trendelenburg gait. Also called waddling gait. The hip swings to the side when a person walks. It can be due to pain, weakness in the hip abductor muscles, or a problem in the hip joint.

ultrasound. Ultrasound uses high-frequency sound waves to look at organs or structures inside the body.

unstable hips. The ball at the top of the thighbone can move out of alignment in the hip socket.

valgus. Outward, away from the center of the body.

varus. Inward, toward the center of the body.

X ray. A form of electromagnetic radiation. In a health-care setting, a machine sends X rays through the body. A computer or special film records the images that are created.

Bibliography

Internet Sources

American Academy of Pediatrics (AAP). "What Is a Pediatric Geneticist?" and "What Is a Pediatric Orthopedic Surgeon?" http://www .aap.org (accessed May 8, 2012).

American Academy of Orthopedic Surgeons (AAOS). "Hip Bursitis." http//orthoinfo.aaos.org/topic.cfm?topic=a00409 (accessed August 5, 2012).

American Association of Orthopedic Surgeons (AAOS). OrthoInfo, "Femoroacetabular Impingement (FAI)." http://orthoinfo.aaos.org /topic.cfm?topic=A00571 (accessed August 5, 2012).

American College of Radiology (ACR) and the Radiological Society of North America (RSNA), Radiology Information: "Arthrography," "MRI of the Musculoskeletal System," "CT Procedures," and "Radiation Exposure in X ray and CT Examinations," RSNA—www.radiolo gyinfo.org (accessed August 5, 2012).

Chen, H. "Arthrogryposis." http://emedicine.medscape.com/article /941917-overview (accessed May 8, 2012).

Children's Hospital at Westmead. "Hip Abduction Orthosis" (Dennis Browne brace). http://kidshealth.chw.edu.au/fact-sheets/care-your -hip-abduction-orthosis (accessed May 8, 2012).

Duke Orthopedics Wheeless' Textbook of Orthopaedics. "Avascular Necrosis Associated with DDH," "Avascular Necrosis of Femoral Head," "Barlow's Test," "CE Angle of Wiberg," "Closed Reduction for DDH," "Developmental Dislocation of the Hip," "DDH 6 to 24 Months of Age," "Femoral Osteotomy in DDH," "Impediments to Reduction in DDH," "Ortolani's Test: for Congenital Hip Dislocation," "Pavlik Harness," "Pelvic Osteotomy for DDH," "Radiographic

Features for DDH," "Treatment of CDH Age 18 Mo to 36 Months," "Treatment of DDH: Newborn (Birth to 6 Months)," "Ultrasound for DDH." http://www.wheelessonline.com (accessed August 13, 2012).

Genetics Home Reference, National Library of Medicine. "Central Core Disease." http://ghr.nlm.nih.gov/condition=centralcoredisease (accessed May 8, 2012).

Hospital for Special Surgery Center for Pain and Preservation. "Periacetabular Osteotomy Guidelines" 2011, and "General Post-Operative Instructions Following Periacetabular Osteotomy," 2011. http://www.hss.edu/physician-files/sink/SinkPAO5.8.12.pdf (accessed January 25, 2013).

International Hip Dysplasia Institute. "Closed Reduction," Femoral Nerve Palsy," "Hip Healthy Swaddling," "Hip Abduction Brace," Impingement," "Open Reduction," "Osteotomy," "Torn Labrum." http://www.hipdysplasia.org (accessed July 9, 2012).

National Institute of Arthritis and Musculoskeletal and Skin Diseases. "Questions and Answers about Osteonecrosis (Avascular Necrosis)." Online version updated October, 2012. http://www.niams.nih.gov/Health_Info/Osteonecrosis/default.asp (accessed January 25, 2013).

Roll Mobility Blog. "How to Load a Wheelchair into a Vehicle," and "How to Push a Wheelchair Up and Down Ramps and Curbs." http://blog.rollmobility.com/2011/02/17/how-to-push-a-wheelchair-up-and-down-ramps-and-curbs (accessed August 24, 2012).

Books

Orthopedic Clinics of North America. *Hip Dysplasia Surgery: Birth to Adulthood.* Vol. 43, No. 3 (July, 2012): 269–408.

West, S., and D. Sutherland. *A Guide for Adults with Hip Dysplasia.* Weston Creek, Australia: Sutherland Studios, 2011.

Journal Articles

American Academy of Pediatrics, AAP Guidelines. "Clinical Practice Guideline: Early Detection of Developmental Dysplasia of the Hip." *Pediatrics* 105, no. 4 (April 2000): 896–905.

Bardo, D. M., M. Black, K. Schenk, and M. F. Zaritzky. "Location of the Ovaries in Girls from Newborn to 18 Years of Age: Reconsidering

Ovarian Shielding." *Pediatric Radiology* 39, no. 3 (March 2009): 253–59. Epub 2009 Jan 8. http://www.ncbi.nlm.nih.gov/pubmed/1913 0048 (accessed January 25, 2013).

Bohm, P., and A. Brzuske. "Salter Innominate Osteotomy for the Treatment of Developmental Dysplasia of the Hip in Children." *Journal of Bone & Joint Surgery American* 84, no. A(2) (February 2002): 178–86.

Eberhardt, O., F. F. Fernandez, and T. Wirth. "Arthroscopic Reduction of the Dislocated Hip in Infants." *Journal of Bone & Joint Surgery British* 94, no. 6 (June 2012): 842–47. http://www.ncbi.nlm.nih.gov /pubmed/22628603 PMID 22628603 (accessed January 25, 2013).

Eberhardt, O., M. Zieger, M. Langendoerfer, T. Wirth, and F. F. Fernandez. "Determination of Hip Reduction in Spica Cast Treatment for DDH: A Comparison of Radiography and Ultrasound." *Journal of Children's Orthopaedics* 3, no. 4 (2009 August): 313–18. Epub 2009 August 6. PMID: 19657686 (accessed January 25, 2013).

Engesæter, I. O., T. Lehmann, L. B. Laborie, S. A. Lie, K. Rosendahl, and L. B. Engesæter. "Total Hip Replacement in Young Adults with Hip Dysplasia," *Acta Orthopedica Scandinavia* 82, no. 2 (April 2011): 149–54. http://www.ncbi.nlm.nih.gov/pmc/articles/PMC3235283 (accessed January 25, 2013).

Frantzen, M. J., S. Robben, A. A. Postma, J. Zoetelief, J. E. Wildberger, and G. J. Kemerink. "Gonad Shielding in Paediatric Pelvic Radiography: Disadvantages Prevail Over Benefit." *Insights Imaging* 3, no. 1 (February 2012): 23–32. Epub 2011 Sep 25. http://www.ncbi.nlm.nih .gov/pubmed/22695996 (accessed August 13, 2012).

Gholve, P. A., J. M. Flynn, M. R. Garner, M. B. Millis, and Y. J. Kim. "Predictors for Secondary Procedures in Walking DDH." *Journal of Pediatric Orthopedics* 32, no. 3 (April–May 2012): 282–89. http:// www.ncbi.nlm.nih.gov/pubmed/22411335 (accessed January 25, 2013).

Grudziak, J. S., and W. T. Ward. "Dega Osteotomy for the Treatment of Congenital Dysplasia of the Hip." *Journal of Bone & Joint Surgery American* 83-A, no. 6 (June 2001): 845–54. http://www.ncbi.nlm.nih .gov/pubmed/11407792 (accessed January 25, 2013).

Holman, J., K. L. Carroll, K. A. Murray, L. M. Macleod, and J. W. Roach. "Long-Term Follow-up of Open Reduction Surgery for Developmental Dislocation of the Hip." *Journal of Pediatric Orthopedics* 32, no. 2 (March 2012):121–24.

Kawaguchi, A. T., N. Y. Otsuka, E. D. Delgado, H. K. Genant, and P. Lang. "Magnetic Resonance Arthrography in Children with Developmental Hip Dysplasia." *Clinical Orthopaedics and Related Research* 374 (May 2000): 235–246.

Luedtke, L. M., J. M. Flynn, G. Stephan, and M. S. Pill. "A Review of Avascular Necrosis in Developmental Dysplasia of the Hip and Contemporary Efforts at Prevention." *The University of Pennsylvania Orthopaedic Journal* 13 (2000): 22–28.

Lerman, J. A., J. B. Emans, M. B. Millis, J. Share, D. Zurakowski, and J. R. Kasser. "Early Failure of Pavlik Harness Treatment for Developmental Hip Dysplasia: Clinical and Ultra-sound Predictors." *Journal of Pediatric Orthopaedics* 21, no. 3 (May–June 2001): 348–53.

Luhmann, S. J., G. S. Bassett, J. E. Gordon, M. Schootman, and P. L. Schoenecker. "Reduction of a Dislocation of the Hip Due to Developmental Dysplasia. Implications for the Need for Future Surgery." *Journal of Bone and Joint Surgery, American* 85-A, no. 2 (February 2003): 239–43.

Mahan, S. T., J. N. Katz, and Y. J. Kim. "To Screen or Not to Screen? A Decision Analysis of the Utility of Screening for Developmental Dysplasia of the Hip." *Journal of Bone and Joint Surgery* 91, no. 7 (July 2009):1705–1719.

Murnaghan, M. L., R. H. Browne, D. L. Sucato, and J. Birch. "Femoral Nerve Palsy in Pavlik Harness Treatment for Developmental Dysplasia of the Hip." *The Journal of Bone and Joint Surgery* 93A (March 2011):493–99.

Price, C. T., and R. M. Schwend. "Improper Swaddling a Risk Factor for Developmental Dysplasia of Hip." http://aapnews.aappublications .org/content/32/9/11.1.full (accessed January 25, 2013).

Price, C. T., "Swaddling and Hip Dysplasia: New Observations: Commentary on an Article by Enbo Wang, MD, PhD, et al.: 'Does Swaddling Influence Developmental Dysplasia of the Hip? An Experimental Study of the Traditional Straight-Leg Swaddling Model in Neonatal Rats.'" *The Journal of Bone & Joint Surgery.* doi:10.2106 /JBJS.L.00297.

Prosser, G. H., P. J. Yates, D. J. Wood, S. E. Graves, R. N. de Steiger, and L. N. Miller. "Outcome of Primary Resurfacing Hip Replacement: Evaluation of Risk Factors for Early Revision." *Acta Orthopaedica* 81, no. 1 (February 2010):66–71. PMID: 20180719.

Russell, M. E., K. H. Shivannna, N. M. Grosland, and D. R. Pederson. "Cartilage Contact Pressure Elevations in Dysplastic Hips: a Chronic Overload Model." *Journal of Orthopaedic Surgery and Research* 1 (2006):6. doi:10.1186/1749-799X-1-6, www.josr-online.com (accessed January 25, 2013).

Sokolovsky, A. M., and O. A. Sokolovsky. "Posterior Rotational Intertrochanteric Osteotomy of the Femur in Children and Adolescents: Use in Residual Deformity of the Femoral Head after Treatment for Developmental Dysplasia of the Hip." *Journal of Bone & Joint Surgery, British* 83-B, no. 5 (July 2001): 721–25.

Steppacher, S. D., M. Tannast, R. Ganz, and K. A. Siebenrock. "Mean 20-Year Followup of Bernese Periacetabular Osteotomy." *Clinical Orthopaedics and Related Research* 466 (2008):1633–44.

Sundberg, T. P., G. A. Toomayan, and N. M. Major. "Evaluation of the Acetabular Labrum at 3.0-T MR Imaging Compared with 1.5-T MR Arthrography: Preliminary Experience." *Radiology* 238, no. 2 (February 2006):706–711. PMID: 16436825.

Upsani, V. V., J. D. Bomar, P. Gaurav, and H. Hosalkar. "Reliability of Plain Radiographic Parameters for Developmental Dysplasia of the Hip in Children." *Journal of Children's Orthopaedic* 6, no. 3 (July 2012): 173–76.

Wang, E., T. Liu, J. Li, E. W. Edmonds, Q. Zhao, L. Zhang, and K. Wang. "Does Swaddling Influence Developmental Dysplasia of the Hip? An Experimental Study of the Traditional Straight-Leg Swaddling Model in Neonatal Rats." *The Journal of Bone & Joint Surgery* 94, no. 12 (June 2012): 1071–77. http://www.ncbi.nlm.nih.gov/pubmed/22573131 (accessed January 25, 2013).

Weinstein, S. L. "Natural History and Treatment Outcomes of Childhood Hip Disorders." *Clinical Orthopaedics and Related Research* 344 (November 1997): 227–42.

Wynne-Davis, R. "Acetabular Dysplasia and Familial Joint Laxity: Two Etiological Factors in Congenital Dislocation of the Hip. A Review of 589 Patients and Their Families." *Journal of Bone and Joint Surgery, British* 52, no. 4 (November 1970): 704–16. PMID: 5487570.

Zielinski, J., G. Oliver, J. Sybesma, N. Walter, and P. Atkinson. "Casting Technique and Restraint Choice Influence Child Safety During Transport of Body Casted Children Subjected to a Simulated Frontal MVA." *The Journal of Trauma Injury, Infection, and Critical Care* 66, no. 6 (June 2009):1653–65. PMID: 19509628.

Resources

This chapter provides additional resources pertaining to hip dysplasia and children's health.

Hip Dysplasia Websites and Organizations

Here are some resources that you might find helpful. Though every effort has been made to select online content that is likely to remain available, the information on websites and their location can change. If you have trouble locating a resource, try a search. Searching is also a good way to discover new information that could have been put online after this list was created. Some key words that you might try are hip dysplasia -canine (using the hyphen tells the search engine to leave out entries related to dogs), clicky hips, CDH, DDH, or developmental dysplasia of the hip.

The following nonprofit organizations offer information about hip dysplasia and online support:

International Hip Dysplasia Institute (IHDI)
1222 S. Orange Ave., 5th Fl.
Orlando FL 32806
www.hipdysplasia.org

STEPS Charity Worldwide (United Kingdom)
Wright House, Crouchley Ln.
Lymm WA13 OAS
England
Help Line: +44 (0) 871 717 0044
Tel: +44 (0) 871 717 0045
www.steps-charity.org.uk/home.php

Support Groups

Hip-Baby is a website with an active online group for parents of children with hip dysplasia—www.hip-baby.org.

Happy Hips is an online group for teens and young adults with hip dysplasia. Happy Hips was founded by a teenager with hip dysplasia—http://happyhips.webs.com

Hip Universe website is a good resource for adult hip problems including hip dysplasia—www.hipuniverse.org.

Integrative Physical Therapy has information about PAO surgery and physical therapy—www.integrativephysicaltherapy.org

Blogs

Abby's Bilateral Hip Dysplasia Story—http://abbysbilateralhipdysplasiastory.blogspot.com

Babies Bulldogs and Us—http://babiesbulldogsandus.blogspot.com

Cameron's Hip Dysplasia Story—http://cameronshipdysplasiastory.blogspot.com

Hip Kid Story—www.hipkidstory.com

One Hip Blog—www.onehipblog.blogspot.com

Hip Kid—www.hipkid.zoomshare.com

Mia's Miracles—www.miasmiracles.blogspot.com

One Hip Baby Mama—www.onehipbabymomma.blogspot.com

Our Tattered Angel—http://aussie-tatteredangel.blogspot.com. This blog and its associated Facebook group is for parents of children who have had surgery for hip dysplasia. The owner of the blog can provide instructions for building a spica chair if requested.

Online Video Resources

Akron Children's Hospital, Patient Success Stories. "Meet Maria: Hip Dysplasia." From this website, search for "Meet Maria" to find the links to a series of videos about a girl who was successfully treated for hip dysplasia. https://www.akronchildrens.org/cms/personal_stories_videos/index.html (accessed August 12, 2012).

Boston Children's Hospital. "Born to Run: How Hip Dysplasia Surgery Got This Patient Moving." (search for Angela McNeeley) May 23, 2012. http://www.youtube.com/watch?v=bShtxYFdERQ (accessed August 5, 2012).

Hospital for Special Surgery. "Hip Arthroscopy Animation." http://www.hss.edu/animation-hip-arthroscopy.htm (accessed August 8, 2012).

Hospital for Special Surgery. "Pediatric Orthopedic Surgery." http://www.hss.edu/pediatric-orthopedic-surgery.asp (accessed August 5, 2012).

Hospital for Special Surgery. "Questions and Answers—Dr. Ernest Sink, Adolescent and Child Hip Specialist and Co-Director of the Center for Hip Preservation, Discusses Hip Pain in Teens and Children." http://www.hss.edu/sink-hip-pain-conditions-teens-children.asp (accessed August 7, 2012).

IHDI Online. The IHDI Online videos show hip-healthy swaddling, questions and answers with Dr. Charles T. Price from the IHDI Medical Board. "Pavlik Harness Application" Part 1 and Part 2, and "How a Child Is Fitted with a Hip Spica Cast." http://www.youtube.com/user/IHDIOnline (accessed August 12, 2012).

Steps Charity has created a number of videos that show how to care for a child in a spica cast. The videos include babies and children in treatment for hip dysplasia, along with their parents. http://www.youtube.com/user/stepscharity/videos (accessed August 5, 2012).

Radiology Info. "Your Radiologist Explains MR Arthrography of the Hip." http://www.radiologyinfo.org/en/photocat/gallery3.cfm?image=kaye_Hip_MR.jpg (accessed August 5, 2012).

Health and Medical Organizations

These organizations provide educational health and medical information or medical equipment. These organizations cannot give medical advice or answer questions about an individual's condition. Contact your doctor with specific questions about your child's personal medical treatment.

American Academy of Pediatrics
141 Northwest Point Blvd.
Elk Grove Village IL 60007
(847) 434-4000
www.aap.org

American Board of Medical Genetics
9650 Rockville Pike
Bethesda MD 20814-3998
(301) 634-7315
http://genetics.faseb.org/genetics/abmg.html

American Board of Pediatrics
111 Silver Cedar Ct.
Chapel Hill NC 27514
(919) 929-0461
E-mail: abpeds@abpeds.org

Automotive Safety Program, Special Needs Transportation
575 West Dr., Rm. 004
Indianapolis IN 46202
(800) 543-6227   (317) 274-2977
www.preventinjury.org

Avenues (athrogryposis support)
P.O. Box 5192
Sonora CA 95370
(209) 928-3688
www.avenuesforamc.com

Centers for Medicare & Medicaid Services (CMS)
Also administers State Children's Health Insurance (SCHIP),
Health Insurance Portability and Accountability Act (HIPAA)
7500 Security Blvd.
Baltimore MD 21244-1850
(800) 267-2323   (410) 786-3000
www.cms.hhs.gov

Easter Seals
230 West Monroe St., Ste. 1800
Chicago IL 60606
(800) 221-6827   (312) 726-6200
www.easterseals.com

Ehlers Danlos National Foundation (EDNF)
3200 Wilshire Blvd., Ste. 1601, South Tower
Los Angeles CA 90010
(213) 368-3800
www.ednf.org

Healthfinder, National Health Information Center
U.S. Department of Health and Human Services
www.healthfinder.gov

In Car Safety Centre, Unit 5 (United Kingdom)
The Auto Centre, Stacey Bushes, Milton
Keynes, MK12 6HS
England
Tel: 01908 220909
When dialing from outside England, you might need to dial an international code first.

National Institutes of Health
9000 Rockville Pike
Bethesda MD 20892
(301) 496-4000   TTY: (301) 402-9612
www.nih.gov; For publications: http://catalog.niams.nih.gov

Pediatric Orthopaedic Society of North America (POSNA)
6300 North River Rd., Ste. 727
Rosemont IL 60018-4226
(847) 698-1692
www.posna.org/index

PubMed
(a free digital archive service of the National Library of Medicine)
www.pubmed.gov

Rhino Pediatric Orthopedic Designs, Inc.
8690 Aero Dr., Ste. PMB-183
San Diego CA 92123
(800) 829-1120   (951) 676-1932
www.rhinopod.com

Safe Kids Worldwide (car seats and restraints)
1301 Pennsylvania Ave., NW, Ste. 1000
Washington DC 20004-1707
(202) 662-0600
www.safekids.org

Shriners Hospitals Headquarters
P.O. Box 31356
Tampa FL 33631

(800) 237-5055
www.shrinershq.org

United Cerebral Palsy Associations, Inc.
1522 K St., NW, Ste. 1112
Washington DC 20005
(800) 872-2827 (Affiliated Relations Dept.)
(800) 872-5827   (202) 842-1266
www.ucpa.org

Special Products and Furniture

Cast Cooler helps to remove moisture from plaster casts—http://cast cooler.com

Hip-Rocker (United Kingdom) features rocking chairs specifically made for children in spica casts—http://hip-rocker.org

IvyRose Spica Furniture offers custom-made chairs with built-in tables designed for children in spica casts—www.ivyrosespicachairs.com

Shrinkins offers removable decorations for casts, crutches, or wheelchairs—www.shrinkins.com

Smirthwaite (United Kingdom) sells hip spica chairs (products, stools, chairs and benches) via their website—www.smirthwaite.co.uk

Books and Booklets

Klapper, R., and L. Huey. *Heal Your Hips.* New York: John Wiley & Sons, Inc., 1999. This book is not specifically about hip dysplasia, but it includes physical therapy exercises that benefit the hips on land and in the water. The exercises are for adults but might benefit some teens.

Patient Advocate Foundation. "Your Guide to the Appeals Process" (free PDF booklet available online). http://www.patientadvocate.org /requests/publications/Guide-Appeals-Process.pdf (accessed August 5, 2012).

Steps Charity has several booklets for families on the subject of hip dysplasia. They are available to download at http://www.steps-charity.org .uk/downloads.

West, S., and D. Sutherland. *A Guide for Adults with Hip Dysplasia.* Weston Creek, Australia: Sutherland Studios, 2011. This in-depth book is the only book in print about hip dysplasia in adults.

Children's Books

These titles are specifically about hip dysplasia:

Craig, L. *One Step at a Time*. This is a children's picture book about a three-year-old girl with hip dysplasia. It is available for purchase at http://www.sandhillbooks.com.

Jay, G., and J. Beattie. *Hope the 'Hip' Hippo*. Altona, Canada: Friesen-Press, 2012. This picture book follows a cheerful hippo named Hope who visits Dr. Kindly to get her hips fixed. Hope wears a spica cast, and the story has some nice, realistic details about the experience. At the end of the book, Hope is back to playing and dancing.

A number of children's picture books are specifically about going to the hospital. You might be able to find a story with one of your child's favorite characters. Here are some children's books about medical topics that might appeal to your child:

Children's Hospitals and Clinics Minneapolis/St. Paul. *A Read-Along Coloring Book*. From the website http://www.childrensmn.org, search for coloring book (accessed August 5, 2012).

Duncan, D., and N. Ollikainen (Illustrator). *When Molly Was in the Hospital: A Book for Brothers and Sisters of Hospitalized Children*. Windsor, CA: Rayve Productions Inc., 1994.

Hopkins Children's Hospital. *A Child's Guide to Surgery Coloring Book*. At the website http://www.hopkinschildrens.org, search for coloring book.

Roy, R. *A to Z Mysteries: The X'ed-Out X-Ray*. New York: Random House, 2005. This is a fun mystery for children from kindergarten to third grade. Can an X ray be a clue?

Health and Medical Articles and Fact Sheets

This section lists articles relevant to hip dysplasia that are written for patients.

Academy of Orthopedic Surgeons (AAOS). "Total Hip Replacement." http://orthoinfo.aaos.org/topic.cfm?topic=a00377 (accessed August 5, 2012).

Agency for Healthcare Research and Quality (AHRQ), U.S. Department of Health and Human Services. "20 Tips to Help Prevent Medical

Errors in Children, Patient Fact Sheet." AHRQ Publication No. 02-P034, September 2002. Agency for Healthcare Research and Quality, Rockville, MD. http://www.ahrq.gov/consumer/20tipkid.htm (accessed January 25, 2013).

American Society of Anesthesiologists, Patient Education Brochures. "When Your Child Needs Anesthesia." http://ecommerce.asahq.org/p-1 45-when-your-child-needs-anesthesia.aspx? (accessed August 5, 2012).

Automotive Safety Program. This website provides information about safely transporting children who are wearing casts. A number of car seats are listed. http://www.preventinjury.org/SNTrestraints.asp (accessed August 5, 2012).

Boba, Inc., Blog. "Strollers, Baby Carriers and Infant Stress." http://www.bobafamily.com/blog/2010/09/20/strollers-baby-carriers-and-infant-stress (accessed August 5, 2012).

Children's Hospital of Philadelphia (CHOP) has a website for children that includes animated characters. http://www.chop.edu/kidshealth galaxy/index.html (accessed January 25, 2013).

Cincinnati Children's Hospital. "Petrie Cast Care." http://www.cincin natichildrens.org/health/p/petrie-cast (accessed August 5, 2012).

Connecticut Children's Medical Center website has information in both English and Spanish about spica casts. See "Home Management of the Child in a Hip Spica Cast" and "Cuidado en la Casa del Niñoa en un Yeso de Cadera Espica." www.ccmckids.org. Search for the name of the article in the website search field (accessed August 5, 2012).

Heisler, J. About.com Guide. "How to Prepare Your Child for Surgery." http://surgery.about.com/od/pediatricsurgery/ss/PreparingPeds.htm (accessed August 5, 2012).

Hospital for Special Surgery (HSS). This website has extensive patient information such as "Family Guide to Pediatric Orthopedic Surgery," "Hip Dysplasia in Adolescents and Young Adults," and "Treatment Options for Hip Pain." Type "hip dysplasia" in the search field or click the "For Patients" tab. http://www.hss.edu (accessed August 5, 2012).

Johns Hopkins Children's Center. Click the "Just for Kids" tab for child-friendly pages such as "My Doctor Visit" and "My Hospital Stay." http://www.hopkinschildrens.org (accessed August 5, 2012).

Kid's Health (Nemours). This website has sections for parents, teens, and children in both English and Spanish. Click tabs on the left or search for the topic that interests you. http://www.kidshealth.org (accessed August 5, 2012).

Phoenix Children's Hospital. See Emily Center. From this website, search for spica cast care. http://www.phoenixchildrens.com.

U.S. National Library of Medicine. Explore MedlinePlus, Medical Encyclopedia, Dictionary, and health topics in many languages. http://www.nlm.nih.gov.

West, S. "A Patient's Journey, Bilateral Developmental Dysplasia of the Hips." *British Medical Journal* 342 (2011):d2152. http://www.bmj.com/content/342/bmj.d2152 (accessed August 27, 2012).

Medical Publications

The documents listed in this section were written for medical professionals such as doctors and nurses. They are presented here for those readers who are comfortable with medical and scientific terminology. To make it easier to locate these publications in Internet searches or medical libraries, they are formatted in a style commonly used to cite medical publications.

Bache, C. E., J. Clegg, and M. Herron. "Risk Factors for Developmental Dysplasia of the Hip: Ultrasonographic Findings in the Neonatal Period." *Journal of Pediatric Orthopaedics B* 11, no. 3 (2002): 212–18.

Berghs, B., N. Wendover, A. J. Timperley, and G. A. Gie. "Impaction Grafting for Acetabular Deficiency in Total Hip Arthroplasty for Developmental Hip Dysplasia." *Acta Orthopaedica Belggica* 66, no. 5 (2000): 461–471. Cited in PubMed; PMID; 11196370.

Berkenblit, S. I., and H. S. Khanuja. "Physician Information, Case Report #7: Total Hip Arthroplasty for Severe Hip Dysplasia Associated with Larsen's Syndrome." http://www.aboutjoints.com (accessed January 25, 2013).

Bobbed P., B. M. Wroblewski, P. D. Siney, P. A. Fleming, and R. Hall. "Charnley Low-Friction Arthroplasty with an Autograft of the Femoral Head for Developmental Dysplasia of the Hip. The 10- to 15-Year Results." *Journal of Bone & Joint Surgery, B* 82, no. 4 (May 2000): 508–511.

Cashman, J. P., J. Round, G. Taylor, and N. M. Clarke. "The Natural History of Developmental Dysplasia of the Hip after Early Supervised Treatment in the Pavlik Harness. A Prospective, Longitudinal Follow-up." *Journal of Bone & Joint Surgery, B* 84, no. 3 (2002): 418–25.

Castelein, R., and M. J. Korte. "Limited Hip Abduction in the Infant." *Journal of Pediatric Orthopaedics* 21, no. 5 (Sep–Oct 2001): 668–70.

Dudkiewicz, I. M., M. Salai, A. Ganel, A. Blankstein, and A. Chechik. "Total Hip Arthroplasty in Patients Younger Than 30 Years of Age Following Developmental Dysplasia of the Hip (DDH) in Infancy." *Orthopedic Trauma Surgery* 122, no. 3 (April 2002): 139–42. PMID: 11927994 (accessed January 25, 2013).

Guile, J. T., P. D. Pizzutillo, and G. D. MacEwen. "Review, Development Dysplasia of the Hip from Birth to Six Months." *Journal of the American Academy of Orthopedic Surgery* 8, no. 4 (Jul–Aug 2000): 232–42.

Hedequist, D., J. Kasser, and J. Emans. "Use of an Abduction Brace for Developmental Dysplasia of the Hip after Failure of Pavlik Harness Use." *Journal of Pediatraic Orthopaedics* 23, no. 2 (Mar–Apr 2003):175–77. PMID: 12604946 (accessed January 25, 2013).

Homer, C. J., et al. "Clinical Practice Guideline: Early Detection of Developmental Dysplasia of the Hip." *Pediatrics* 105, no. 4 (2000): 896–905.

Lehmann, H. P., R. Hinton, P. Morello, J. Santoli, Committee on Quality Improvement, and Subcommittee on Developmental Dysplasia of the Hip. "Developmental Dysplasia of the Hip Practice Guideline: Technical Report." *Pediatrics* 105, no. 4 (April 2000): E57.

Martus, J. E., and D. J. Sucato. "Developmental Disorders of the Hip Age 0–8 Years." *Current Opinion in Orthopaedics* (renamed *Current Orthopaedic Practice – A Review and Research Journal*) 18, no. 6 (November 2007): 529–35.

Mubarak, S. J., F. G. Valencia, and D. R. Wenger. "One Stage Correction of the Spastic Dislocated Hip: Use of a Pericapsular Acetabuloplasty to Improve Coverage." *Journal of Bone & Joint Surgery* 74A (1992): 1347–57.

Rab, G. T. "Pediatric Orthopedic Surgery." In *Current Diagnosis and Treatment in Orthopedics*, 2nd ed., ed. H. B. Skinner. 532–76. New York: Lange Medical Books, 2000.

Ruhmann, O., D. Lazovic, P. Bouklas, S. Schmolke, and C. H. Flamme. "Ultrasound Examination of Neonatal Hip: Correlation of Twin Pregnancy and Congenital Dysplasia." *Twin Research* 3, no. 1 (March 2000): 7–11.

Vitale, M. G., and D. L. Skaggs. Review, "Developmental Dysplasia of the Hip from Six Months to Four Years of Age." *Journal of the American Academy of Orthopedic Surgery* 9, no. 6 (Nov–Dec 2001): 401–11.

Wall, E. J. "Review, Practical Primary Pediatric Orthopedics. Developmental Dysplasia of the Hip Section of Pediatric Orthopaedics." *Nursing Clinics of North America* 35, no. 1 (March 2000): 95–113. In *Essentials of Musculoskeletal Care*, 2nd ed., ed. W. B. Greene. 630–33. Rosemont, IL: American Academy of Orthopaedic Surgeons, 2001.

Weill Cornell Medical College, Cornell MRI Laboratory Group. "MR Imaging, Hips: Routine Protocol." 2008. http://www.med.cornell.edu /mri/MRI/Pelvis/Hip_protocol_files/Hip.htm (accessed August 5, 2012).

Yaster, M., and S. Kost-Byerly. "Acute Pain Management in Children." http://www.nysora.com/regional_anesthesia/sub-specialties/pediat ric_anesthesia/3088-acute_pain_management_in_children.html (accessed August 22, 2012).

Index

Italicized page references indicate illustrations.